THE WAYS OUR BODIES AGE

THE WAYS OUR BODIES AGE

THE PHYSIOLOGY OF AGING

KATHERINE R. SCHLAERTH, MD

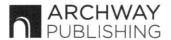

ARCHWAY PUBLISHING

Archway Publishing books may be ordered through booksellers or by contacting:

Archway Publishing
1663 Liberty Drive
Bloomington, IN 47403
www.archwaypublishing.com
844-669-3957

Because of the dynamic nature of the Internet, any web addresses or links contained in this book may have changed since publication and may no longer be valid. The views expressed in this work are solely those of the author and do not necessarily reflect the views of the publisher, and the publisher hereby disclaims any responsibility for them.

Any people depicted in stock imagery provided by Getty Images are models, and such images are being used for illustrative purposes only.
Certain stock imagery © Getty Images.

ISBN: 978-1-6657-6941-9 (sc)
ISBN: 978-1-6657-6942-6 (e)

Library of Congress Control Number: 2024925721

Print information available on the last page.

Archway Publishing rev. date: 01/28/2025

C O N T E N T S

CHAPTER 1

Aging demographics, theories, projections....and the individual!

Overview of the aging process: Statistics and projections about present and future generations

Mrs. T woke up early one morning and looked at her skin in the cold light of the morning sun streaming through the bedroom window. It used to be a deep ebony color, but now it was tending more towards milk chocolate. Then her gaze turned to her snoring husband. Time was when he'd be awake ahead of her, and at the first sign that she was approaching consciousness, would be ready for an early morning round of lovemaking. Her gaze shifted to the pictures on her dresser. Their six children, in Sunday best, four boys and two girls. Right alongside that picture was another in which the couple's fifteen grandchildren were lined up by height, the two babies in the teenagers' arms. What a family reunion that had been!

Mr. B didn't have a picture in his bedroom to remind him of happier times. When his wife died, he'd exiled all their photographs to her old cedar chest. Looking at a picture of her, holding their two little boys, was just too much. The children were doing well, married and with offspring of their own. He seldom saw or heard from them though, because they both lived about 3000 miles away, one to the North and the other to the South. Travel was impossible. He couldn't lug the suitcases, and the grandchildren barely knew him anyway. When his wife was alive, skyping was a ritual every weekend. But now as he looked at his loose yellowish skin, balding pate and drooping jowls, he felt the grandkids might be frightened by his appearance.

The world is aging fast. People are having far fewer children than in times past, primarily because offspring don't have the economic value they did in the heyday of farming and cottage industries. Then too, sexual intercourse has become dissociated from its generative function. On the other side of the equation, individuals are surviving all over the world, into what was once considered extreme old age. The reasons are many, but the widespread introduction of public health measures including vaccinations, improved access to cleaner water and more secure food supplies, and perhaps a recent reduction in pandemics (excluding Covid, of course) could be part of the reason. Think of bubonic plague, which devastated Europe and Asia in the fourteenth century, the influenza epidemic of 1918 which killed more humans that WWI, and the carnage that infectious diseases like smallpox and measles inflicted upon Native Americans who had never been exposed to these lethal maladies before. In 1900, a little over 4% of the population was older than 65, and only two in a thousand lived past 85. Now days, almost 17% of folk have passed their 65th birthdays, and ten times as many people live to age 85 as did over a century ago. In 2060, it is projected that almost a quarter of the population will be over 65 and one in twenty will have almost exceeded their allotted fourscore and seven year life span. (1) (the World Almanac, 2019) Unfortunately, with aging comes a boatload of problems. As long ago as 2013 statistics indicated that about a quarter of individuals over 65 had difficulty ambulating, over 10% couldn't easily get out of bed or even a chair, and once people had passed their 85th birthdays, half couldn't walk.(2) (Chapter 1-Demography, Paul Scarzo, BS and Luigi Ferrucci, MD, PhD. Geriatric Review Syllibus, 9th edition. Editors-in-Chief: Annette Medina-Walpole, MD, AGSF, James T. Pacala, MD, MS, AGSF and Jane F. Potter, MD, AGSF.) All of these statistics boil down to one fact: society must evolve ways to deal with the anticipated "Elder Boom" and older persons must maintain function for as long as possible.

In fact, one of our states is already dealing with this youth implosion-elder explosion. Poor old Maine, way up there in the cold Northeast, is certainly no Florida attracting tons of retired folk. One third of its population is over 60. Nursing homes and in-home care is just not available to meet the needs of these older people. Many who qualify for care cannot get any. It just isn't available! The other side of Maine's quandary is that there are not enough young workers to fill regular jobs, let alone provide care for a growing and aging population.(3) (Jeff.stein@washpost.com)

Historical perspectives about aging

Everyone has heard the theory of aging in paleolithic times. Grandma, whose rheumatism was too severe to permit her to move with the rest of her hunter-gatherer kin following the herd, was left on the tundra with a chunk of meat and a small fire. Pretty quickly the animals would come and make a meal of her. This scenario may well have happened in some times and places among our primordial ancestors, but our knowledge of aging in remote historic times is mostly conjectural. Mark. E Williams, MD, a geriatrician, suggested that ancient Greeks who prized "youth and vigor" may have been somewhat lukewarm to the aging process, but did prize wisdom and experience, especially in Sparta. In anticipation of one current theory of aging, that of the loss of telomeres, many Greek thinkers including Hippocrates and Aristotle, postulated a diminution in one's innate heat or vital force which slowly leaked away as an individual grew older. (Telomeres are nucleotide sequences at the end of chromosomes which protect the integrity of the chromosome, but with repetitive DNA replication, the telomere shortens. One theory of aging is that this gradual shortening causes aging)

As for ancient Rome, older persons apparently could participate in activity as their stamina permitted and were excluded from certain duties as they grew frail. One legendary hero of the Roman Republic, Cincinnatus, was said to be an older man working on his farm when he was called to rescue Rome in a time of crisis. Having defeated the evil Aequi and rescued a portion of the trapped Roman army, he went back to his farm. Much of his story is probably highly embellished. A gentleman doing family research, was astounded to discover that his 18th century ancestors, peasants and workers in middle Europe, lived till their 80's.

The United States has always been a youthful country. Irish, German, Asian and most other immigrants left their parents behind in the old country. Once here, the immigrants had many children, and died young themselves. In 1900, males at birth could expect to live 46 years and females 48. If you were African American however, your life span would be 14 years shorter than that enjoyed by your Caucasian brothers and sisters. This gap has narrowed to under four years today, and in 2016, both Blacks and Whites could expect to live well into their seventies.

Aging in different cultures

Most cultures consider aging in a slightly different light. In most parts of Central and South America, older folk live with their families and often assume domestic responsibilities as they are able. A lovely lady from Mexico, during a casual encounter in a store checkout line, told of how she traveled daily to another city to care for her three grandchildren while their parents worked, and her husband did the same for another grandson in yet another town. The weekend would bring an influx of still more relatives for whom she would cook traditional cuisine. Asia is a composite of many different cultures, and Japanese citizens have the longest lifespans in the world. Both China and Japan are facing a huge cultural crunch due to low birth rates. China's one child policy meant that one grandchild would be shared by four grandparents. Chinese tradition holds that the most well-situated child must care for parents. Most often, this was a son, perhaps the eldest. This custom becomes practically impossible for families to sustain when four aging grandparents must lean on one couple. China has recently allowed families to have two offspring. In Africa, again a mix of many cultures and languages, generalizations are difficult . However African families are usually fairly large, and the lifespan of Africans in general is rising rapidly. In many sub-Saharan cultures, grandparents are also an integral part of the family.

In most cultures, the elderly have traditionally been a source of wisdom, and help with childrearing, their evolving frailties accepted as a part of the web of life. Such an approach may change rapidly as the internet envelopes everyone, and an older person's wisdom may not extend to the use of new technologies.

Changing societal attitudes towards aging

The more rapidly technologic evolution takes place, the more aging folk may feel themselves out of place. A recent small nonpublished study done by some resident physicians indicated that older folks' ability to use facets of electronic communication like skyping or twitter depended both on their education and on their employment status. No community resources were easily available to teach those who wanted to learn about computers.

Many older folks no longer have families to interface for them. Birth rates have more than halved from as recently as 1960 to the present, while divorce and infertility rates have soared. Almost as many women as men are working. No-one is left at home to care for poor spinster Aunt Sally.

Social Security became law when most people didn't live much beyond 65. Now this underfunded mandate is expected to be the main source of sustenance for ten or more years for most mature folk. Imagine how a young adult with student loans is going to feel when his taxes must also support a burgeoning senior population!

Some older persons are acutely aware of this. Widowed Mrs. O, for example, cares for disabled older neighbors, doing their wash and shopping. This relieves the state from the cost of institutionalization. Mr. T makes it his business to drive the sick elderly in his neighborhood to their medical appointments. Mr. Z does all the carpentry and repair work his church needs. Over four and a half million Americans over 65 remained in the work force paying taxes in 2018.

The aging individual's perspective

The S's are an active couple. Hovering around age 80, both are active in sports, live in the home where they raised their five children, and enjoy neighbors who have aged vigorously with them. However, the couple are adamant about not being a burden for their children or thirteen grandchildren. To this end, they have looked into assisted living, burial issues, wills and other messy business associated with getting really old.

Mr. J is 75, divorced, with children he still hangs out with. A skilled motorcycle mechanic, he works from home, and loves a good ride in the mountains every weekend.

Mrs. F, a traditional Asian mother, lives with her daughter's family and looks after the four children when needed. However, she is getting frailer. Tasks that are becoming too difficult are now done by others.

Mrs D relied on her youngest son to care for her, discouraging any romantic attachments he seemed to be forming. Imbued in the culture of the "old country", she felt that his life was owed to her care. She died in her eighties, and her lonely son died a year or so later, still a bachelor.

Mr S, visiting his parents in Florida, went to a church service where the elderly congregation all arrived about 15 minutes early. He quipped that they were all waiting for "the bus to heaven" and didn't want to miss it.

Clearly, there are many ways of looking at the aging process. Attitudes reflect culture, a desire for both independence and for closeness with others, and issues of function. However, certain attitudes seem more universal. These include reviewing and evaluating one's live and accomplishments, a certain pride in one's offspring if any, often a renewed attachment to one's religious beliefs, and a desire, often elusive, for closeness with other human beings.

Why do we age?

Have you ever planted roses, and watched changes as the summer season evolved? Each rose buds, blooms, grows old, and finally is autoamputated from the bush, to be replaced by another group of buds. An old Native American saying, incompletely articulated, suggests that we must grow old and die so that new humans can have their chance to be born and grow.

Theories of aging are diverse and not too helpful practically speaking. However, here are a few, abbreviated in a way that probably doesn't explain their complexity.

Evolutionary theory holds either that after reproduction ceases, mutations accumulate over time, and because an organism is no longer reproducing, there is no evolutionary benefit one way or the other to cull bad mutations from the evolutionary pool. Another theory holds that a gene which may improve reproductive fitness may do the opposite and decrease fitness as aging occurs

Psychosocial theories look at adaptability to changing environments and duties as we age.

Physiologic theories get down to the nitty gritty of cell structure and function. They examine cell and mitochondrial DNA, the aforementioned telomeres, and delve into epigenetics. Mechanisms of damage may extend from free radicals through metabolic rate and on to radiation. (4) (Neal S.Fredarko, PhD, Matthew K.McNabney, MD, AGSF in Chapter 2-Biology. Geriatric Review Syllabus, 9th edition, American Geriatric Society, 2016, Annette Medina-Walpole, MD, AGSF, James T. Pacala, MD, MS, AGSF and Jane F. Potter, MD, AGSFR, Editors-in Chief)

In essence, we don't really know exactly why everything from trees to bobcats age, and perhaps all theories have some truth, much like the allegory of the six blind men and the elephant, found in Buddhist, Hindu and Jain texts.

Fitting into society, and the roles played by seniors here and elsewhere

If you come from Asia, Africa or South and Central America, you will be honored for your wisdom, and cared for as best the family can. You will be expected to contribute what you can towards the family, perhaps caring for grandchildren, cooking and cleaning, and even advising on family issues. In current Europe and upper North America, excluding migrant and more traditional groups, you and the state will assume the bulk of your care. Your impact on your biologic family may be less intense. Of course, there are so many evolving exceptions to these generalizations, that they are more historical than accurate in most cases and depend very much on the individuals and family constructs involved. For example, if you, like Dr. C, started a dental practice, and your daughter joined your practice upon graduation from dental school, chances are that your influence will be quite pronounced!

Giving back to society, and "not being a burden"

Mrs. T was coming up on eighty-five, was a bit forgetful, and lived alone. She was an endless frustration for her only child and his wife. Clearly, she could not safely look after herself. However, she would not allow the hiring of a person to help her with her daily activities, constantly berated her family for their concerns about her safety, but still depended on them to help her out whenever she got into a jam, which was often. There was no reasoning with her, and she denied being a part of any conversations addressing her wellbeing.

Contrast her with Mrs. H, a longtime widow whose children were a part of her life on holidays but whose life's work was being the neighborhood go-to person for rides, a meal during episodic illness, or perhaps being a volunteer at a church fundraiser.

Every community offers opportunities for seniors to "give back" and lots feel a moral obligation to do so. Even Mrs. k, who into her nineties would knit booties and sweaters for babies whose mothers were disadvantaged financially.

Isolation and loss

Statistically speaking, widows and widowers are at an increased risk of dying. There is even an entity called "widower's syndrome" in which a man whose wife has died may become impotent in a new relationship. In psychologic terms, his impotence occurs because it seems to be an abandonment of fidelity to his deceased wife.

Loss is a constant threat to older persons. A spouse dies, a friend moves into a nursing home, children live across the country. Add to this insult, an ongoing reduction in physical appearance and ability. In fact, in 2010, over 25% of people in the USA lived alone…and many were elderly!

Preparing communities for worldwide aging: chronologic vs functional aging

One of the issues gerontologists look at is what is called the activities of daily living. These include bathing, feeding oneself, toileting, dressing, even getting out of bed and combing one's hair (if any) or shaving. Instrumental activities of daily living encompasses cooking, taking medications, using the telephone, shopping, driving or taking public transportation, paying bills and in the near future will probably involve using a computer! There are ninety-year-olds who manage all these activities well, and fifty year olds who do not. One's years are not a good measure of one's functional abilities!

Creating a community where functional capacity will be maximized is the task of the near future. This humongous task will fall to city planners, architects, government officials, even geographers and weather forecasters. It will vary from community to community and reflect the values and cultures of those involved.

Social and work responsibilities of seniors: maximizing contributions

Our current culture doesn't really utilize the skills of the older person. In fact, many people complain that being hired if one is over 50 is, in some industries, almost an impossibility! However, other occupations are handicapped when a senior worker retires. For example, one engineer was overheard lamenting the retirement of so many talented and experienced individuals in a profession where life experience is possibly more important that educational degrees! The engineers and scientists who got us to the moon are old now, and their experience is currently irreplaceable! The age at which one is eligible for social security is advancing, but in the future, people will have to stay in the workforce longer to make up for the lack of replacements. Perhaps the good news is, as a research article in Gerontology and Geriatric Medicine from 2015 concludes, "Being gainfully employed, having a higher level of education, and being physically active in their leisure time reduced the chance of presenting disability (in seniors)" (5) (Paid Work and Physical Activity Preserve Functional Capacity in Elderly People", Laraine Mortean Ono, MMSc, et al. Gerontol.Geriatr Med, 2015. Jan-Dec1. Published online 2015, Sept 23)

Living in a rapidly evolving world with new technologies

Perhaps the most difficult challenge for folks is mastering new technology. Everything from buying a new winter coat to looking up one's ancestors is on the internet. Currently, health care demands a working knowledge of so-called "Patient Portals". In this new age of Covid 19, even doctors' appointments are often done through telemedicine encounters. The challenges of mastering new technology, with no chance to get instruction in the nuts and bolts of this technology, can keep a person up at night! We know there are sensitive periods in one's life for learning new skills. Those learning periods occur abundantly in two-year-olds, but have all but vanished in eighty-year-olds. Nonetheless, the brain is a remarkable instrument, even in old age. New neuronal connections can be made. It just takes much longer and must be mated with a driving desire to learn new skills and having the resources to do so. Two forces oppose keeping up with the times. One of these forces is internal. One often hears the viewpoint that paradise will come when retirement age approaches. Retirement becomes one's goal in life and is conceived as a time of indulgence and leisure. The second force is external. Opportunities simply don't exist to master new skills. Illness can take a toll too. Arthritic hands don't text very well. There is a huge need for technologic advances to incorporate specifications that will allow older folk and disabled individuals access to electronic communication and other burgeoning technologic changes.

Facing philosophic, demographic, religious and even product changes as one ages

"The children now love luxury; they have bad manners, contempt for authority; they show disrespect for elders and love chatter in place of exercise. Children are now tyrants, not the servants of their households. They no longer rise when elders enter the room. They contradict their parents, chatter before company, gobble up dainties at the table, cross their legs, and tyrannize their teachers." (Socrates, ancient Greek philosopher)

Country music lovers may remember Alan Jackson's classical song, "Remember when" from almost three decades ago, which seems to tell the story of young love, parenthood, struggles and good times from a long-ago perspective. Things always look better in the rear-view mirror, because the rough spots in life are somewhat smoothed over by time, and the good times similarly magnified by time. Back in the day, African Americans were treated as second class citizens, and sometimes feared for their lives just for being in the wrong place at the wrong time. (Unfortunately, this is still true today, and not just for those of African ancestry). Televisions measured about 10 inches and were black and white, songs were written about the frustration some women felt being suburban, stay-at-home mothers, but things were still better than they were in the preceding generation. Back three or four generations, employment opportunities sometimes carried the caution that "no Irish need apply". Electricity and plumbing were not guaranteed, automobiles were a rare luxury, and most children had two pairs of shoes if they were lucky. The Great Depression made our current recessions look like child's play.

However, as we age, the old ways of doing things takes on a soothing familiarity. Normal changes in products, religious practices, even the disappearance of the comics section from childhood (where did Dick Tracey and the Katzenjammer kids go?) can bring a sense of disassociation leading to depression. Most aging people deal with change well, but some do not.

Becoming a demographic minority as one's, generation slowly thins

Although persons over 65 are becoming a larger percentage of society, older folk are still a minority overall. Old age brings a decline in the ability to get out and do things. One widow in her seventies who badly wanted to travel acknowledged that she couldn't find any contemporaries with her sense of adventure to globe-trot with her. Another family bragged in their annual Christmas card that they were still strong enough in their mid-seventies to drive all over the East Coast, hike and camp out! Not too many contemporaries seen along the way! Older folk with computer skills may look at their Facebook or Twitter accounts perhaps a couple of times a year. Usage of all forms of communication between distant friends seems to drop off significantly somewhere in the early to mid-seventies.

What matters most as one ages

What seems apparent is that familiar landmarks, from people to products, slowly drop out as persons age, and need to be replaced with the new. Perhaps that is why religion (irrespective of one's belief system) and family assume so much more importance. It does take energy to stay current and energy is the one thing that seems to dissipate parallel with the aging process.

Learning potential in the elderly

Older people who are retired seem to be motivated to learn new material because they are interested in the subject matter and because learning can be a platform for social interaction. (6). (Ahjin Kim and Sharan B. Marrian: Motivations for learning among Older Adults in a Learning in Retirement Institute. Educational Gerontology, Vol.30, Issue 6, 2004.) WE know that people who remain physically and mentally active in their senior years also remain healthier. In addition to motivation, the capacity to learn new material remains present in aging rats and aging humans. Given that learning can occur in older adults, and that motivation is a big part of learning, and given the corollary that older folk will of necessity have to participate more in formal or informal work to keep society above water, a lot of work will have to be done in the future to make that happen. Educational programs may have to adjust to the unique learning speed and sensory needs of older learners who want to continue in their professions or reestablish an employment toehold. Hidden prejudices about aging and learning will have to be unlearned by society.

Educational attainment in youth and its impact on learning in the senior years

Almost fifty years ago, a young researcher named David Snowden, decided to study a group of nuns to see how their brains aged. Nuns, as everyone knows, live under similar environmental circumstances, and usually have entered religious life in their teens or early adult life. The nuns, at the time of entrance to religious life, were asked to write an essay, or autobiography, which was analyzed by Snowden for the cognitive ability of each nun-writer in her youth. What was found was that researcher, many decades later, could often predict which nuns would go on to have dementia just from reading those early essays. It seems that nuns who had written less idea-rich and complex essays as young women were more likely to develop dementia, and even to have shorter lives than those who had a richer thought life. These nuns were also the ones who got more education while in the convent and were likelier to teach as part of their vocation. The study continues but does emphasize that ongoing cognitive involvement throughout life reduces the risk for dementia.

Many older people immigrating from Mexico have had only a second-grade education. That, of course, has changed in more recent times! However, the range of cognitive ability in older persons who have started with minimal education is startling. Some have taught themselves English, and mathematics, have mastered reading and developed writing skills, while others have lost what little literacy they possessed.

Given the evidence of the need for lifelong learning of all sorts, an aging society needs to encourage learning activity across the age span, just to keep its senior citizens healthy and productive!

The effect of the availability of resources on the ability to adapt

Everyone knows the old saying, "Give a man a fish and he will eat for a day, teach him how to fish and he will eat for a lifetime". Our research has shown that in one important area, the ability to communicate electronically, many older persons, especially those who speak Spanish, just don't have the opportunity to learn how! Classes aren't available, computers and cell phones are expensive, arthritic hands are not nimble. Nowadays, so many resources are primarily available electronically that the need to acquire computer skills is urgent!

Meeting this and other needs, while involving older persons in productive societal activity becomes more urgent as births decrease and longevity increases worldwide.

We are going to need everyone from city planners to car designers, from clothing manufacturers and designers to providers of gardening supplies, from frozen food manufacturers and nutritionists to companies that produce lightbulbs and lamps, to get on board, learn a bit about the challenges and opportunities presented by a growing elderly population, and provide us with the opportunity to make seniors productive and healthy members of their respective societies.

Nor are seniors off the hook. There is the obligation to maintain health through exercise and healthy eating, the duty to stay current with skills, stay away from bad foods and bad drugs (yes, substance abuse is a problem for older people too!!) and decrease screen time in favor of interacting with others.

And we must make these course changes in the way society views aging quickly! The crisis is already upon us…worldwide, and not just in Maine!

CHAPTER 2

Changes in the Sensory Organs

Normal changes in vision with aging

Mr. A had a very successful life, considering the obstacles that he had faced at birth. He was born with club feet at a time when a poor boy would just have to endure this birth defect. He was also not the sharpest kid on the block, and no-one in the early 20th century thought about special education for kids like him. But despite poverty, mild retardation, and a permanent gait disorder, he managed to support himself through his adult years working as a janitor.

In his golden years, he ended up in supervised senior living, a happy content guy. Then something happened. The supervisor at the facility, a kindly "father stand-in" for his aging seniors, noticed that Mr. A was falling quite a lot. Putting together Mr. A's congenital foot issues with the falls, the supervisor decided that some corrective foot surgery was in order, so off Mr. A went to his geriatrician. The physician agreed on a referral to an orthopedist, but Mr. An emphatically dd not. However, Mr. A would permit surgery on his newly identified cataracts. After having just one eye corrected, Mr. A's falls stopped completely. Mr. A had a longstanding acquaintance with using his clubfeet safely, but the cataracts were new and the real cause of his falls.

Structure and function of the eye

The eye is a superb organ. From front to back, its construction meets the needs of an intelligent biped. The cornea, a clear window in the front of the eye, is bordered by the white sclera, a protective membrane, and behind the cornea is the lens, which focuses light onto the nerve of the eye which lines the back of the globe called the retina. The retina's job is to convert light rays into electrical impulses subsequently transmitted to the optic nerve. These impulses eventually get to the occipital lobe of the brain and become our vision or sight. The eye being a globe, with the cornea and lens anterior and the retina in the back of the globe, there are two liquid components, one between the cornea and lens (aqueous) and the other behind the lens (vitreous) which give shape, and in the case of the aqueous, nourishment to the adjacent eye structures. The aqueous exits from the space between the cornea and lens through a strainer called the trabecular network. Which if blocked can cause a very dangerous buildup of pressure in the front eye.

The retina itself is an engineering wonder. It is a sensing lining of the back and sides of the globular eye, containing photoreceptors called rods and cones. Cone cells are responsible for color vision and are concentrated in the macula, the retina's central area. Rod cells are located mainly in the peripheral retina and their job relates to peripheral vision, night vision and detection of motion.

The eye needs protection. Tears, produced in the lacrimal gland of the upper eyelid, lubricate the eye when we blink. The eyelids and eyelashes protect the eye from too much light and from other external agents like dust. The eye itself is nestled in a protective semicircle of bone.

The complexity and importance of the eye and its attachments make it vulnerable to some specific diseases that usually occur with advancing years. Some of these diseases and natural changes progress so slowly that a person may not even be aware of any visual loss!

Timing of normal changes of aging

Mr. B, an architect, was only 43, and in the office for his yearly physical, which he managed to get done about once every five years. This year he was quite concerned. He and his wife had just welcomed their third child, a baby girl. Three children to send through college, and his eyes were already giving out! How could he pursue his profession, when his near vision seemed to be diminishing to the point where he had gotten some cheap lenses to be able to read architectural "blueprints" at work.

Our eyes undergo predictable changes as they age. Mr. B had presbyopia, part of the normal aging process where the eye's lens loses its normal flexibility. Loss of flexibility and lens elasticity makes it harder to focus on things like the printed word, or the small writing on maps. Near vision is affected most and by fifty years of age, nearly everyone has encountered this problem. Those at most risk are persons who are farsighted and surprisingly, persons who live at sea level or in tropical climates! Luckily, there are many remedies, from eyeglasses through LASIX.

Other eye symptoms are attached to presbyopia such as needing brighter light to see well, feeling "eye strain" leading to headaches, increased sensitivity to glare, and decreased night vision. Luckily presbyopia, although progressive, seems to stabilize in the seventies.

The why and what of vision changes

With regard to retinal ganglion (nerve)cell death, we lose, it is estimated, about 5000 axons a year which translated, means about ½ percent of the nerve cells in our eyes. The damaged cells are mostly in the area of the retina where glaucoma also occurs. Coupled with presbyopia, normal changes of aging will cause significant vision issues in an older population.

The effects of diminishing vision on seniors' daily functioning

Visual loss, meaning visual acuity of less than 20/40 affects a quarter of the population above 75. Two percent are legally blind. Add to this the other changes of aging in the eyes and elsewhere, and seniors can be significantly affected in ways that may not even be immediately apparent .

With an increased need for more intense light, seniors may not be able to drive well in the dark. Decreased peripheral vision may mean bumping into people or things, hogging walkways without realizing it and having problems driving when other vehicles approach from the side.

Gardening may be an issue, as bumps in the ground or steps may not be seen. Using small screen computers, smart phones and other modes of communication may be too much work for people with diminishing eyesight. In fact almost every aspect of daily living depends on sight! Couple this with the fact that problems with vision may creep up so slowly that seniors are not even aware of their handicap, and you have a recipe for everything from falls to dinner preparation without key ingredients!

Common eye diseases that occur as we age

There are a number of eye diseases that uniquely plague seniors and pre-seniors, and several of these have genetic, ethnic and racial proclivities that demand our awareness.

Cataracts are lens opacities that reduce vision. Half of individuals over 75 have cataracts. These and refractive errors like nearsightedness (myopia. Very popular among students), farsightedness (hyperopia) and distorted vision (astigmatism) are the leading cause of visual loss everywhere.

Age related macular degeneration causes most irreversible blindness in the developed world. This eye disease has genetic, environmental and age-related roots and is commonest in Caucasians, especially very pale-skinned ones. Age related macular degeneration has two subtypes, dry and wet. The dry form doesn't usually cause many visual problems. It is identified by drusen, yellow plaques or spots in the retina that are markers for the evil wet form where blood vessels grow where they shouldn't and obstruct central vision. People who have wet macular degeneration have poor central vision, needed for reading and doing things like sewing and texting.

Glaucoma hits African Americans especially hard. It is the leading cause of blindness in black Americans and the second leading cause worldwide. Though there are many forms, slow drainage of aqueous fluid from the anterior chamber of the eye, the area between the cornea and the lens, is most common causing increased pressure in the eye leading to decreased peripheral vision. Functionally it is somewhat the opposite of macular degeneration, which hits central vision and affects reading and similar activities. Glaucoma doesn't let one see the margins of vision, and visual changes can creep up so slowly that the individual doesn't even notice something is wrong. There once was a lively African American lady of ninety or so years. She had gone blind from glaucoma unrecognized until it was to late. However, she kept a beautiful vision in her memory, of a field of yellow sunflowers she had seen as a youth. This old memory became her consolation for her current loss of vision, as she could always see it in her "mind's eye" when her loss of vision saddened her.

Diabetic retinopathy

Diabetic retinopathy is the curse of people with longstanding diabetes and one of the reasons people with diabetes are constantly hounded by nurses, physicians, dieticians and daughters to control their eating and check their blood sugars at home every day. Diabetic retinopathy damages the retina, that part of the eye which translates things we see into electrical impulses that travel to the visual cortex of the brain allowing us to "see". Diabetic retinopathy can cause macular edema (the macula being the most precise seeing part of the eye)or macular nonperfusion (no blood flow to nourish the macula).

Neovascularization (blood vessel overgrowth) and proliferative diabetic retinopathy can be associated with hemorrhage and traction macular detachment (pulling the macular retina from its functional position in the eye).

What medical remedies are available?

Cataracts are amenable to surgical treatment. Taking the cataract lens out surgically and replacing it with an artificial intraocular lens which can also be selected to eliminate refractive error (farsightedness, nearsightedness and distorted vision) can lead to amazingly better vision and the surgery is easy even for elderly folk with other medical problems. For refractive errors by themselves, glasses are usually safer and better received than lasik.

Age related macular degeneration if "dry" demands close follow up for high risk drusen deposits on the retina. Additionally, high dose oral multivitamin/mineral therapy is used to retard or prevent progression especially to "wet "macular degeneration .

The "wet form" of macular degeneration with sudden onset of vision loss or distortion is a medical emergency. A breakthrough in treatment of "wet" macular degeneration is the injection of vascular endothelial growth factor, into the vitreous of eye. This retards the wild damaging growth of those blood vessels (neovascularization) that eventually cause the central blindness associated with wet macular degeneration.

Other new medications in are also recently available and can be used by ophthalmologists.

Glaucoma needs to be looked for in vulnerable people through screening every 1-2 years in those over 50. African Americans, persons with a family history of glaucoma may need more frequent screening. Eye drops or other medications which either decrease production or increase outflow of that buildup of aqueous fluid in the anterior chamber of the eye can stop pressure buildup and progressive reduction of peripheral vision. For people who cannot use eyedrops or other medicines, a procedure called laser trabeculectomy opens the drainage system of the anterior eye and prevents ongoing damage.

Diabetes is uniformly a major threat to health, and diabetic retinopathy is just one aspect of this big problem. Again, damage to the retina is the biggest threat to vision, so in addition to controlling blood sugar and blood pressure, regular eye exams are very important to find and treat retinal changes early. Treatments range from laser photocoagulation to more complex surgery and even anti-vascular epithelial growth factor injections (see macular degeneration) to stop aberrant blood vessel growth have helped prevent blindness.

Other eye problems have other remedies, but the important aspect of preserving vision and therefore independence is regular eye exam and recognition of abnormal or progressive vision loss, often by those around the senior if not the senior herself.

How to avoid or delay vision loss

In addition to regular eye exams, knowing one's family history well is important in recognizing and preventing specific eye diseases. For example, knowing one's mother developed glaucoma in her fifties would make a pre-senior start regular glaucoma checks even prior to that age, and look for possible symptoms. Blood pressure control would also be important in this and other eye diseases. One lady in her forties, whose mother had just been diagnosed with macular degeneration, decided to start taking the over-the-counter vitamins and minerals recommended for possible delay in symptom onset, although it should be remembered that care must be taken to prevent very high amounts of fat soluble vitamins which also can cause illness. Checking with one's health care provider would be prudent in these cases.

Preventing diabetes, through healthy eating and regular appropriate exercise and especially blood pressure control is a very important, though difficult intervention. Seniors should have yearly ophthalmologic exams to spot early disease.

Altering the environment for persons with eye issues

Recognition of visual problems and adaptation of the environment can prevent falls and the loss of ability to care for oneself.

The "walkthrough"

One important task that can be done by anyone, but especially occupational therapists and others with special training is the home "walk through". One lady in her late seventies had several falls, and one forearm fracture. Her physician in this case did a home visit and found stacks of newspapers dating back 20 or 30 years all over the home. Other obstacles could range from throw rugs to poor lighting.

An older person with visual problems may be aware of and able to avoid the obstacles in her own home. When visiting relatives and others, her vision problems may be riskier. An eighty something lady with wet macular degeneration did well in her own small apartment. Her daughter in law was terrified of the risks of a visit. Small children, toddlers and toys created all sorts of obstacles not present in the mother in law's home.

Assistive devices

These ay range from quad canes to walkers and even wheelchairs and may be needed only in risky environments and especially if vision problems occur side by side with proprioception or gait issues.

Obstacle mitigation

This endeavor can be done in one's home, or on a larger canvas, may involve architecture which considers problems with vision and other aging changes. An architect, for example, may construct a health center with wall bars for elderly patients to hold on to, furniture may be positioned to give a clear visual path from one room to another, and lighting may be of higher intensity and with reduced glare. Number of steps may be reduced and well-marked, and elevators installed which have wheelchair capacity. Windows allowing for natural sunlight and strategically positioned may also be a cheerful way of increasing the intensity of light which seniors may need to see better.

Use of color and design

Reduced vision of whatever cause is improved by lighting and bright contrasting colors. Steps can have alternate colors, for their horizontal and vertical components. Each wall in a room may also be painted in contrasting but tasteful color. Glass doors need something on them to show the glass is present! Architects and interior designers can be very helpful in designing living space for those with restricted vision

Smell, the most primitive sense

Before the eye and brain developed in living organisms, there was a sense of smell. Lancelets, creatures that diverged from our ancestors 700 million years ago, had olfactory or "smelling" genes There are actually two categories of genes for smell: one for marine creatures to detect odors in water, and the other for airborne odors.

Animals have varying smell acuity based on their environmental use of smell for survival. Dolphins, for example, have a smaller subset of genes for smell. Animals who use their eyes and ears as survival tools also need less olfactory power.

Physiology and neurology of smell

Newborn babies can recognize their own mothers by smell, and even prefer Mom's smell to other people's smells for the first few months of life. Unfortunately, as we age, the sense of smell may variably decline and with it, the ability to appreciate life-threatening odors like fire and rotten food. How does this ancient sense work anyway?

Smell organs, called the olfactory mucosa, are located in the upper part of the nose, along structures located laterally called the turbinates . You can see these structures when you look up through the nares, those openings at the base of the nose through which air enters. These smell receptors are also located in the upper nasal septum. The surfaces of these receptors boast a mucous layer producing secretions which also contain infection fighting agents like immunoglobulins, lactoferrin and lysozymes. Odorant binding proteins transport odor molecules to receptors.

These olfactory chemoreceptor cells are actually neurons that go through to the brain and are formed repeatedly during adulthood. Cilia, which are hairlike projections from the neurons, have receptors or mooring apparatus, which bind the "odorants". The axons (Long slender projections from the nerve cell, AKA nerve fibers)of the above mentioned neurons travel through a structure called the cribriform plate and collect, all 10-20 million of them, to form the olfactory nerve in the brain

After this feat, nerve pathways then journey with their smell information to the olfactory cortex, orbital frontal cerebral cortex, thalamus and hypothalamus. Essentially smell information is distributed to several parts of the brain.

Some Covid 19 victims have described a loss of smell. The reasons for this attack on the nose and possibly the nervous system are unsure, but will be undoubtedly explored!

The part played by smell in survival

Since smell has evolved over so many millions of years and has adapted to the environmental circumstances in which life forms find themselves, it has to be important for survival. Persons who run in the dark or in remote locations will testify to the fact that they can pick up on the presence of animals which should be avoided by smell. Pheromones, which are chemicals secreted by animals ranging from insects to ourselves, stimulate a social response in others of the species. These responses may evoke alarm, transmit feeding information, or even engender affection. They play an important part in reproduction.... presumably even in humans!

Mammals such as dogs, cats and many others, will urinate on the turf they consider theirs, to warn other animals away. Smells can warn of danger, spoiled food which should not be eaten, gas leaks, burning items. The list is huge and can be species specific too. Affection for infants is undoubtedly enhanced by their sweet smells (unless they need a diaper change) Memories are evoked by smell. One lady, who didn't remember much of her early childhood, had a portion of memory unlocked by sensing an odor that she'd only been exposed to many decades before, when her long deceased soldier-father carried her into a "hole in the wall" restaurant with the same smell..

The sense of taste

Taste buds have a reputation that far exceeds their prowess. When we say that food tastes good, we inevitably dismiss the colossal part smell plays in our gustatory pleasure.

Taste buds are much simpler anatomically than the olfactory apparatus They are located on top of and on the lateral parts of the tongue, but also hang out on the soft palate, uvula, throat and even down to the esophagus (AKA food tube). There are around a hundred, more or less, taste receptor cells within each taste bud, but these taste receptor cells have a short life, lasting only about ten days. Taste receptor cells connect to neurons, and the conversion of taste into neural information (transduction, a complex process)) occurs at this intracellular level.

There are three types of tongue papillae, wherein dwell the lingual taste buds. The fungiform papillae hang out on the anterior 2/3 of the tongue, being most plentiful at the tip of the tongue. The foliate papillae are located on the posterior sides of the tongue. The circumvallate papillae are in the back of the tongue. Three distinct nerves innervate the tongue, and so testing different parts of the tongue can identify what connections are affected by neurologic disorders. Of note, saliva plays an important role in getting food and other molecules to the taste buds. This means that changes in quality or quantity of saliva, for example with an autoimmune disease like Sjogren's which can cause a dry mouth, can lead to malnutrition due to swallowing difficulties as well as lack of interest in poor tasting food.

Taste buds can pick up on four, perhaps five taste qualities. These include sweet, sour, salty and bitter. A fifth, called umami,, (glutamate) has been identified too.

Loss or diminution of the sense of smell: consequences

A 60–something year old African American lady was beside herself. She had a bad sinus infection, and when it resolved, she noted that she no longer had a sense of smell. Food was tasteless, several specialists had been consulted to no avail, and life took on shades of grey when she couldn't enjoy her own culinary productions. So she stopped cooking.

A 64-year-old Filipino man, already distressed by medical problems which had put him on disability, was attempting to make a meal for his wife when she returned from work. Unfortunately, he had become somewhat forgetful, and had lost his formerly satisfactory sense of smell. His wife, on arrival home, recognized immediately that there was a gas leak and an unattended stove. Her tongue lashing was nothing compared with the response of his daughter, who returned home a few minutes behind the wife. The sad part of this story was the response of the unfortunate man. His comments that he was useless reflected both his failure to turn off the stove, but more significantly, his feelings of worthlessness now that he was no longer the breadwinner and family protector.

What about the loss of smell and taste with aging? Deficient smell on testing affects about 1 person in 4 of those more than 70, but rises to over 1 in 3 in folks over eighty. Seniors who can't smell their food, since smell is the most important aspect of food appreciation, will often decrease intake. When that happens, malnutrition with all its attendant risks supervenes. In an effort to make food palatable, seniors who are losing taste bud function as well, will over-salt their food, or excessively sweeten items, which doesn't help if they already have diabetes and/or hypertension!

Hearing and balance

Although the following cautionary tale is about one marriage, similar tales could be told of many marriages in many cultures, and in many eons. Mrs. X and Mr. X had lived together in Holy Matrimony for four and a half decades and had prospered. The usual reefs upon which marriages shipwreck had been by-passed. Mr. X never had a midlife crisis because he was too busy providing for his five children to covet a new red convertable or woman. Mrs. X glossed over the empty nest syndrome because her nest never completely emptied. When the last child left for college, his place was immediately taken by a new grandchild whose working mother needed a reliable babysitter.

Then came the biggest challenge of all. Mr. X retired. Mrs. X gritted her teeth when Mr. X rearranged all her kitchen cabinets. She understood his need to be productive when he uprooted and replanted her herb garden. But his lack of communication was driving her crazy.

So, off the couple went to their Parish priest (Rabbi, Iman, minister, shaman, therapist) for marital counselling. She said "He never listens to me. The house could be on fire and I could be shouting for him to leave, and he would keep on reading his darn paper (making his darn arrowheads, whittling his darn wooden boats)" He said "She is always mumbling. I can't understand a word she is saying".

Luckily for this couple, the Minister, Rabbi, Iman, Shaman, therapist or Priest was quite familiar with this common marital problem . The solution was not so simple, however. Mr. X had no desire to wear a hearing aide, because it was an outward sign of aging. Mrs. X needed to turn down the TV and speak very distinctly in a low tone. Spontaneous conversation became difficult, so compromise about when to use the hearing aid was needed too. Divorce avoided!

Hearing problems can be very isolating and can even lead to depression. They do increase with age, also with a prior history of exposure to ambient noise, and men seem more affected generally.

The gyroscope and the snail inside your inner ear: How they team up for hearing and balance

To understand the ubiquity of hearing problems, a brief description of the complex structure of this sense is in order. The ear of course is not just an organ of hearing. Balance is also integral part of the cochlea, the organ converting sound and position into impulses conducted by the auditory nerve to the brain.

Sound waves are funneled by the pinna, the part of the ear we see, through the external ear canal, to the tympanic membrane or "eardrum". When sound waves hit the eardrum, they cause it to vibrate, and the vibrations are transferred to three little bones in the middle ear, the malleus, incus and stapes, also known as ossicles. The stapes abuts on a structure called the oval window, a part of the cochlea which bridges with the semicircular canals. This is where it all happens.

The cochlea looks a bit like the shell of a snail and is connected to the semicircular canal which resembles a gyroscope via the vestibule, which houses the saccule and utricle.

The semicircular canals contain fluid called endolymph and fine hair cells. When you move, or even tilt your head, the fluid moves, stimulating the hair cells in the saccule and utricle, and through a complex process the hair cells convert the perception of movement into electrical impulses traveling through the vestibular nerve to the brain. In the brain, these signals from the inner ear are coordinated with signals from the optic nerve and the skeletal system to maintain balance and coordination. This process will be important in looking at the causes of dizziness and falls in the elderly.

Meanwhile the snail -like cochlea is also sitting in the inner ear, connected by the vestibule with the semicircular canals, and ready to take on its task of converting sound vibrations from the three bones of the middle ear into nerve impulses to be sent to the brain again through the auditory nerve. It does this conversion once again through the medium of cochlear fluid and hair cells.

You can see that a lot can go wrong between the collection of sound waves by the pinna (external ear) and their interpretation by the brain.

Male vs female hearing

Changes include thinning of the walls of the ear canal and drying out of cerumen or ear wax. It is not uncommon to have a senior in clinic whose complaint on not being able to hear is completely resolved by disposing of the wax in the external ear canal by means of a wash-out " bath". The ear drum loses its shiny thin appearance and becomes thickened and there is loss of hair cells and neurons in the cochlea. There are other changes in the structure of the hearing apparatus, but probably one of the more interesting occurred in the brain's sensory auditory processing. Did you know that as a young right handed adult, your right ear has a 5-10% advantage over your left ear, but if you are eighty something, that advantage goes way up to almost 50%?

For some reason being a genetic male increases the possibility that you will lose hearing earlier. Loss of hearing at higher frequencies is associated with exposure to noise. One gentleman, in the process of herding his five screaming, fighting young children, commented that he was sure he would go deaf by the age of sixty. But be aware that if you are Black, statistically you will have better hearing as you age.

Along with the normal changes noted with aging, some quasi-pathologic conditions are common among older folk. Sensorineural hearing loss usually reflects damage to the cochlea, due to aging itself or to heredity, vascular disease, and even medications which can damage hearing. If you are a non-smoker, and live in a quiet rural area, and your occupation has not involved exposure to noise, you will probably maintain your hearing acuity longer. Presbycusis, literally translated as "older hearing", can be caused by cochlear pathology, by brain difficulties or by both. An audiogram can be helpful for evaluation.

Persons with sensorineural hearing loss may initially have difficulty hearing in places like restaurants where there is a high level of background noise. One-on-one they do fine. As problems advance, there is difficulty with high pitched sounds. Finally, normal conversation has attendant difficulties.

Besides presbycusis and other cochlear issues, and cerumen impaction, other conditions can cause poor hearing. Middle and outer ear infection, eardrum perforation, fluid in the middle ear from allergies or a viral "cold", otosclerosis (changes in those little ossicle bones in the middle ear), and cholesteatoma (a clump of skin debris in the middle ear) are among other common causes of hearing problems.

Determining the cause of a hearing loss involves an inspection of the outer and middle ear, an audiogram which tests for hearing at different pitches and levels of sound intensity, and possibly imaging as indicated. Audiologists and otolaryngologists are specialists instrumental in doing evaluation and instituting therapy for hearing problems.

Some of the consequences of not hearing well that you may encounter

Social isolation is a frequently encountered problem as people age and spouses and friends become ill or die. Add to this the monetary, health and transportation problems some seniors deal with and social isolation becomes a real possibility. If on top of other difficulties, people cannot hear well, isolation seems inevitable! This isolation can lead to depression, because we remain social beings even as we age, and lack of someone to talk to can be a real "downer". Similarly, if persons cannot hear, a sense of paranoia can set in. We are all somewhat egocentric even as we age. Lack of ability to hear what others are saying while at the same time seeing them talk, can translate into a suspicion that unkind things are being said about us!

Many aspects of safety, from telephoned community warnings through hearing a car coming towards us as we walk, are transmitted through sound. If you can't hear the telephone ring, the water steaming on the stove, your grandchild screaming, you are at risk for accidents or worse.

And let's not forget interpersonal and marital problems. Intimacy is not helped by hearing difficulties, but many a spouse or older parent is reluctant to use a hearing aid, either due to cost, or the mis perception that such an instrument increases others' estimates of the wearer's age by ten years.

Clues to recognizing a hearing problem

One non-native speaker of Spanish noted that if senior patients had difficulty understanding her imperfect but passable Spanish, it was probably because they had an incipient hearing issue. This became her unscientific screening test for ear issues

However, there are several other clues to poor hearing, and all can easily be missed. Many elderly persons are not aware of their poor hearing because it happens slowly. Their families may recognize signs such as turning up the TV or the radio to a noise level which annoys other, not responding to a question posed by someone out of view, misinterpreting questions or statements, or even seeming to have early signs of dementia. In new settings, classically with hospitalization, hearing loss may present as delirium or may be associated with it.

There are questionnaires which allow the senior to give information about his or her hearing. For example, the Hearing Handicap inventory for the Elderly-Screening version has ten questions inquiring into what problems the senior may be experiencing in day-to-day activities due to imperfect hearing. If you are looking for an easy, quick way of validating your suspicion of less that pristine hearing, try the whisper test. Stand two feet away from a person who has occluded one ear and whisper a series of numbers and letters. See if the subject can feed it back to you. For detailed precise instructions, the University of Nebraska Whisper test is accessible on the internet.

If you know a senior is hearing disabled and doesn't have a hearing aid, and you must interview that person, here are some suggestions for more effective communication. First, ask the senior if he has tips for communicating more effectively. Get his attention, sit where he can see your lips and expression, have good lighting and make sure the room is quiet. Speak slowly and distinctly and if possible, at a lower pitch. Separate your words for more clarity. The patient may identify a "good ear" so focus sound on this ear. If you need to, write words, spell them, and ask the person to tell you what you just said to be sure he has received the information correctly. If the patient speaks another language as his first language, a native speaker in that language may be helpful.

What is proprioception?

Have you ever been in a store check-out line and watched with increasing frustration as an elderly lady has tried with limited success to separate the bills to pay for her items?

Or have you observed an elderly man's attempt to shuffle the pages in a book?

Perhaps you have stood behind an elderly person in a checkout line and watched with amusement as that person's trunk swayed a bit more that your own body even though both of you were standing patiently still in line waiting to pay for your respective purchases.

Proprioception is a difficult sense to define, and usually operates in conjunction with the other senses.

It is the sense of the relative positions of body parts and also of the degree of effort needed to move these body parts. Specialized nerve endings are involved in eliciting data from joint capsules, tendons and muscle and transmitting this data so that we know, even without using other senses, where our limbs, for instance, are in space. However, proprioception usually is teamed with other neurologic input. For example, the lady in the checkout line and the gentleman opening pages are relying on their sense of touch and on vision as well as where and what the muscles, joints and tendons in their fingers and hands are doing.

Proprioception is an interesting "sense" that we use every moment in our daily activities without even realizing it. Our own actions stimulate the above nerve endings, and they are a part of, and collectors of information for, whole groups of afferent nerves, which are outgoing nerves taking information to the central nervous system, the spinal cord and brain. These afferent nerves inform the central nervous system of where the trunk and limbs are in reference to each other and to the environment and what movements they are enacting. You can see those muscles, joints, tendons need this sense of proprioception on a continuous basis to monitor and modify their function. Muscles, joints, tendons etc., through the afferent nerves of proprioception feed information to the brain, which in turn, and usually with input from other senses like vision, sends outgoing messages to the tendons, muscles and joints for them to modify their activity to realize a goal. When you want to take a step, your afferent or outgoing nerves, having plugged into the muscles, joints, tendons of your lower extremities, tell the brain where your legs and feet are and then outgoing nerves, having gotten directions from the brain, make the muscles, joints, tendons contract in a way that will allow you to take the next smooth step. When you are walking, of course, you don't just use proprioception, your inner ear is also feeding the brain with balance information, and your eyes and nerves of touch are transmitting directions about the surface you are walking on, about obstacles in your path and your "tiny grey cells", as the detective Hercule Perrot would say, are also cognating about where you are going and why.

Proprioception and motor function are intimately joined together and assisted by all the other senses. Decrease in proprioception occur with aging but may also be magnified by aging changes in other senses.

As an aside, proprioception is not limited to systems involved in movement. We also have receptors for distension in arteries, lungs and gut. These are receptors, that tell us we are gassy or bloated, for example.

Getting back to our little old lady trying to isolate the five-dollar bill in her purse from all the other bills, or the grandfather attempting to turn to the next page of the book he is reading to his grandson, a decline in proprioception isn't the only issue. The sense of touch comes into play too.

WE have lots of nerve receptors in our skin. Some skin areas are more abundantly gifted with sensory receptors that others. To understand touch and the changes that occur in this sense as we age, it is important first of all to know a bit about the structure of the skin. There are two main layers in the skin, the epidermis or top layer and the dermis or bottom layer. Immediately underneath these layers is fatty tissue. Getting back to the skin itself, the dermis is the top layer and is thicker in some areas like the palms and soles. The bottom layer, called the dermis, is where the action is. The dermis houses our hair follicles, our sweat glands, and sebaceous glands (oil glands) and unlike the epidermis, has blood vessels

The nerves of sensation come in different flavors too. Sensory nerve receptors exist in skin muscle and joints. Large, sheathed nerve fibers carry proprioceptive, vibratory, pressure and touch information and smaller poorly sheathed nerve fibers are responsible for pain, temperature and touch sensations. Some of the nerves of the skin begin in the epidermis and some in the dermis. The large and small nerves carrying pain, temperature and touch information end up in the spinal cord, where they relay information to (or synapse with) other neurons (nerves) going up through the spinal cord to the thalamus, a brain structure, where they unload sensory information (touch, pain, temperature) to yet another set of nerve cells going to the primary sensory cortex of the brain. This long journey occurs rapidly and finally upon arrival in the brain itself, nervous information collected in the skin and other structures enters our consciousness. Manifestations of this sensory information can present as sensations we use daily. For example, two-point discrimination allows us to be aware that two distinct stimuli are touching different parts of our skin at the same time. Try this on yourself. Touch your palm with two fingernail tips from your opposite hand. How far do the fingernail tips have to be apart, eyes closed, before you appreciate them a s two different stimuli? Or in that old child's game, have someone write letters on your back and see if you can identify the letters.

What happens to these skin senses as we age?

Skin structure changes, of course, with thinning of the outer layer, or epidermis, loss of elasticity atrophy of skin structures like melanocytes which if not lost, produce less melanin which gives skin its traditional color. We also have fewer hair follicles and those we have turn grey, not just on our heads either! Our skin has immune cells and reparative cells, and these also become less plentiful and less active.

An 89-year-old lady demonstrated these changes when she took out a bag of trash to her curbside garbage can. Unfortunately, a shard of glass from a broken container worked its way through the plastic garbage bag and caused a superficial cut above her ankle. A teenager could have sustained the same injury and not needed to seek medical attention at all. However, this poor lady was brought to the clinic and started on antibiotics after wound cleaning. Two days later, despite appropriate antibiotics, she had developed a cellulitis (deep skin infection) and had to spend the weekend in the hospital getting wound care and intravenous antibiotics. Her skin defenses were so weakened by the changes of aging that antibiotics by mouth weren't sufficient to reverse the infection after the cut.

But when we are talking about the effect of aging on the skin's sensory function, atrophy of skin structures is only one facet of the problem. The peripheral and central nervous system plays a big part too. Brain volume decreases and the functioning of the remaining sensory neurons (nerves) declines. Neurons transmit information more slowly, so reaction time to a stimulus increases. Not good if you are touching a hot stove! Nerve cells communicate with each other by appendages called axons and dendrites, and these grow more slowly. Then we need to consider the damage that conditions and diseases of aging can cause to nerves.

Mr. A was a very noncooperative patient. He had diabetes for at least a decade, but advice from physicians didn't stop him from eating fast foods and consuming sodas daily. To be fair, his wife was incapacitated and Mr. A didn't know how to cook. He noticed numbness in his feet, especially in the night. He soon felt as though, as he described it," I was walking on hot sand and pebbles". He had a peripheral neuropathy, with damage to the nerves of his feet from his poorly controlled diabetes.

Other conditions that can cause peripheral neuropathy include vitamin deficiencies such as lack of vitamin B12. Loss of sensation in older folk, like a similar loss in younger people, needs to be fully investigated, but meanwhile, caution needs to be taken to avoid damage or falls due to the person's inability to recognize painful or pressure stimuli.

CHAPTER 3

Bones and muscles: Why is exercising so difficult these days?

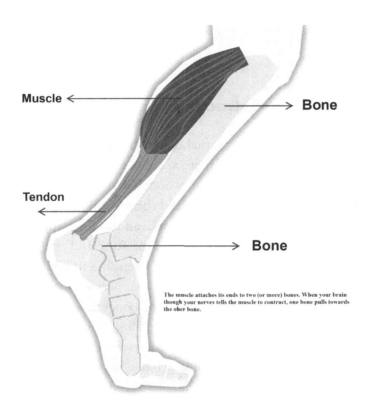

Muscle ← → Bone

Tendon ←

→ Bone

The muscle attaches its ends to two (or more) bones. When your brain though your nerves tells the muscle to contract, one bone pulls towards the oher bone.

Problems with bones, muscles and joints are probably as old as mankind. Take, for example, Grauballe Man, found in a bog in Denmark. He died roughly around the late 3rd century BC, and somewhat violently, it appears. The bog preserved his body well, so we can tell that the poor guy died at about age thirty and already had arthritis of his spine.

Anasazi women, living in the Southwest US about a millennium ago, whose lives centered around grinding corn or maize to make food for their families, seemed to have a lot of arthritis, based on studies of their skeletal remains.

In fact, even dinosaurs had arthritis, usually the gouty type, but a 70 million year old Hadrosaurus from of all places, Appalachia, was identified as having a septic, or infectious, arthritis of its radius and ulna, or upper limb.

Yet bone and joint problems tend to cause the most trouble in older humans. Bones and joints affected can often vary based on heredity, also by occupation, by type of arthritis, and even by diet! The problems caused by malfunctioning bones and joints not only make older folk miserable but

25

can also domino into other diseases. Take, for example, the diabetic who can't exercise because of wear and tear knee arthritis. It will be more difficult for such a person to control her diabetes, because using one's muscles really helps to lower blood sugar and even cholesterol. Having elevated cholesterol and blood sugar will put a diabetic at risk of other problems like heart disease and even foot infections with their complication. It is obvious that minimizing arthritis symptoms is significant in a multitude of ways.

Muscles and the motor component of the nervous system

To understand the complexities of motor function, we first need to look at the structure and also the mechanics of muscles.

How muscles and nerves are structured and how they function together

Muscles, attached to bones by ligaments, make those bones move by contracting and thereby pulling on the bone to change its position. There are about 700 or more muscles in the human body, and they should make up about half of a body's weight......unless we become couch potatoes, or grow older and don't move as much, and then fat takes over.

There are three types of muscle. The heart is a muscle, and additionally there is smooth muscle, found in the walls of structures like the stomach and intestine and responsible for the forward propulsion of food and finally, waste. These muscles have some intrinsic ability to contract on their own and are also under the control of the autonomic nervous system. They do their thing involuntarily and under the influence of a variety of hormones and other substances.

When discussing movement, however, we are referring to skeletal muscle, a collection of striated muscle fibers interwoven with and surrounded by connective tissue or "fascia", attached to bone by tendons, fed and stimulated by capillary blood vessels and nerves branching within the muscle fibers which make up the entire muscle. . Each individual muscle fiber ultimately has its very own nerve. The strength of a muscle is determined by the its cross-sectional area and by the laws of physics applying to its leverage. Tendons, which bind the muscle to bone, are bundles of collagen fibers, very strong in youth. WE often encounter adolescent athletes, whose bones have not yet fused completely, and whose tendons are so much stronger than muscle and unfused bone, that in running or repeatedly* jumping to make a basket, can tear off a small part of bone attached to those strong tendons. IF this happens in the knee, there will be a big bump over the shin bone. The name of this condition is jumper's knee or patellar tendonitis. In the heel, the problem is called Sever disease and makes running painful.

Normal aging changes in the motor unit consisting of muscle enervated by nerve

Most older people lose muscle mass from disuse and subsequent infiltration of fat and connective tissue into the muscle itself. This age-related loss of muscle strength and volume is called sarcopenia. Seniors lose strength in their legs more so than in their arms. Initially, at least in men over fifty, the number of individual muscle fiber units decreases and so does innervation. Some people suspect that the loss of nerve fibers contributes to the loss of muscle fibers. Expect the handshake from a thirty-year-old man to be on average about twice as strong as that of an analogous 80-year-old man. (7) (George E. Taffet. MD. In Normal Aging, Jan.9, 2017, Up to Date, Kenneth E. Schmader, MD section Editor, WWW.uptodate.com) Tendons also become weaker and more likely to rupture under stress

One sixty-year-old couch potato decided to play some basketball while on his island vacation. Something snapped and he came into the local clinic in pain and with a malfunctioning left foot. He had torn his Achilles tendon, that big tendon that goes from the calf muscle to the heel, ending his vacation and replacing it with a visit to a mainland orthopedic specialist.

Common muscle complaints in the elderly

When a woman has a pap smear, she is placed on the exam table in what is called a lithotomy position, lying on her back and with legs separated in stirrups. This position is necessary in order to place a speculum in the vagina and gain access to the mouth of the uterus, called the cervix, for cell scrapings. It is an unpleasant procedure, but one which will allow the identification of abnormal cells. These rogue cells almost always harbor a nasty virus called the human papilloma virus, which over time can cause cancer. Eliminating the rogue cells with their infecting papilloma viruses can save many lives. However, the lithotomy position often causes strong leg cramps especially in overweight older women. Leg cramps are not limited to women having pap smears. Mature men and women, stretching in bed or doing other motor activities, will get a "charley-horse" in their legs, toes or even elsewhere which can be very painful and can interfere with sleep.

Another bothersome type of muscle pain is called restless leg syndrome. People will complain of an unpleasant sensation sometimes described like having ants crawling up and down one's legs. Constant movement, not consistent with getting a good night's rest, gives relief. Although children can be affected, and need testing for iron deficiency, most sufferers are older adults, and can be helped after an evaluation for contributing factors. The medications giving relief happen to be those commonly used for Parkinson's Disease.

Then there is the spinal column. Pinched nerves, caused by narrowing of the places in the spine where nerves exit from the spinal cord, can affect the muscles served by these nerves. Sciatica is a prime example. The sciatic nerve travels down the leg, so a "pinched" sciatic nerve with cause pain running laterally down the affected leg.

Gelling is a common complaint, especially when a senior has been in one position, such as being seated, for a while. It is just difficult to get muscles and joints going. Everything feels stiff. Once one gets moving, things improve remarkably.

Common and not so common diseases of muscles and nerves

Most people have heard of Lou Gehrig's disease, Lou Gehrig being a Yankees baseball player almost a century ago whose courage merited naming the disease scientifically called amyotrophic lateral sclerosis after him. This degenerative condition involves motor neurons, generally lower ones first, followed by upper . People start with symptoms, like falls, foot drop, gait disturbances that can mimic other problems of aging, so this can be a difficult disease to pick up early in its course.

A while ago, a sixty-year-old complained of increasing weakness in one leg and the opposite arm. After much probing, he gave a remote history of paralytic polio, from which he recovered completely as a child. The limbs affected in childhood were the same ones weakening as he aged. Post polio syndrome involves dysfunction of the surviving motor neurons, and then of the muscles served by these motor neurons. It usually occurs decades after recovery from the initial bout of polio. Fortunately, polio vaccine has been in use for about sixty years, so this disease should soon disappear.

Consider the case of Mrs. M. She had Graves' Disease, caused by too much thyroid hormone. Besides her loss of appetite, depression and general withdrawal from the activities she loved (Seniors guild at church, making cookies with grandkids), the big clue leading to the treatment of her overactive thyroid was the fact that she was having increasing difficulty climbing the stairs to her bedroom. The muscles of her upper arms and legs were atrophying (losing tissue) due to her excessive thyroid hormone production.

There are many more diseases which involve the nerves and muscles, but muscle weakness needs to be investigated, leading as it can to falls, problems with daily activities and a host of other issues

What are tendons, bursae, ligaments and how do they work?

Complex interrelationships between joints, muscles, tendons, bursae etc

First, some definitions. Joints are places where two or more bones meet. Some joints such as the knee or shoulder joints allow for a good deal of motion, and others, like the sacroiliacs where the pelvis links up with the spine, allow for little movement. To function appropriately, joints that are made for movement need to do so smoothly. Bursae are the ball-bearings of the body. They are sac-like structures containing synovial fluid that allow tendons and muscles around a joint to glide over each other . A tendon is that thick band of fibrous tissue that connects muscle with bone and transmits the force of the contracting muscle into movement of the bone to which it is attached. Ligaments are fibrous tissue that attach bones to bones . Cartilage is firm but resilient tissue that cushions bones. Joint fluid allows bones such as those in the knee, a hinge joint, to move easily over each other.

Changes in these structures with aging

The cartilaginous connective tissue lining of joints, especially of the knees, spine, hands and hips, can thicken and synovial tissue become inflamed due to years of hard use. Bones are no longer protected by cartilage and synovial fluid so they can rub against each other. The subsequent inflammation and damage can extend deep into bony structures. Osteophytes, which appear like bony drippings off the involved bone itself, can form. So, the bones of your joints, without their protective cartilage and lubricating synovial fluid, will make movement more painful. The natural response to pain itself is not doing whatever activity causes the pain. Unfortunately, this withdrawal from painful movement results in muscle wasting, because muscles must be used if they are to function well. Strong muscles also support joints. So the perfect vicious cycle of muscle disuse, wasting and lack of support develops. Add to this mix the fact that tendons and ligaments shorten and become less flexible, and you have a recipe for joint replacement surgery. However, physical therapy, stretching exercises, and getting muscles to do their job again can minimize pain and delay the need for surgery.

Strains, sprains and bursitis

These events are not unique to the elderly but can happen to anyone. A sprain or strain is damage to a ligament or tendon by forceful stretching beyond the normal range of function. Ankle sprains are common examples. Bursitis is irritation and inflammation of one of the bursal sacs, either from trauma or even from infection. Unfortunately, healing usually takes longer the older one is.

Mrs. TT had discomfort in her right hip. It caused her pain when she inadvertently rolled onto her right-side during sleep. She became convinced that her right hip would need replacement. Her doctor examined her and noted tenderness over the olecranon bursa of the right hip, reassuring her that since her hip x-rays were normal this problem too would pass with a little help. And it did.

Common problems in hips, knees, neck, back, shoulders

Wear and tear changes in joints and their appendages, and even disuse make musculoskeletal complaints some of the most common seen by providers.

Mr. T had been a football player in high school and college, we won't say where, but he did attend a powerful football university. Upon graduating, he took a sedentary business job, got married, had two children, developed a social life with its share of business dinners. Exercise wasn't on his personal radar, though it should have been. His weight slowly accelerated. Now in his late forties, he was having some serious hip discomfort. Unfortunately, years of microtrauma followed by years of disuse and weight gain had made him vulnerable for early arthritic changes. Joint replacements, depending upon the material used, have a limiting shelf life. His orthopedist was interested in putting off surgery for a while.

Mrs S, an immigrant from a less advantaged country, now had four teenage and young adult children and a husband who did construction when jobs were available. She had worked in a local hotel as a maid for decades, lifting, cleaning showers, making beds and pushing heavy carts. It was steady work, helped pay the bills, but her left shoulder was starting to give her a lot of pain when she made beds and had to reach up high to clean the bathroom mirrors in the hotel rooms. At night, she would wake in pain when rolling on to her left side. One particular area that can sustain overuse damage earlier than other sites is the shoulder's so called rotator cuff. The shoulder is a magnificent joint. The three bones involved, the clavicle in front, scapula in the upper back and the humerus, the bone of the upper shoulder, glide beautifully around each other and allow us to do things with our arms and hands that no other creatures, not even members of our genus, are capable of. The shoulder joint is held together by a whole assortment of ligaments, tendons and bursae, which attach to various sites in the chest and neck. The shoulder is a truly remarkable feat of engineering! However, we also use our arms a lot. Macro and microinjuries to the structures in the shoulders, including partial and complete tears, are common even in early to mid-adulthood.

Mrs. J, a rather large lady to begin with, had almost doubled her weight over the course of raising her children, and becoming the grandmother of three rug rats. Her knees caused her a lot of pain, and then one day she tripped over a curb in the parking lot where she worked. That did it. X-rays didn't show any fracture, so she probably had just sustained a sprain. However, x-rays did demonstrate severe knee arthritis so bad that the middle areas of both knees were "bone on bone". Mrs. J quit her part time job after her fall, got a quad cane, later replaced with a walker, and settled into a life of eating and watching TV. Her diabetes got worse, and no orthopedist would replace her worn out knees until she lost some of her now massive girth. The story does end on a slightly more optimistic note. Mrs. J was seen by several specialists at a world-famous university medical center, started to take her health more seriously, so her weight gain ceased as her diabetes stabilized. She didn't get her knee replacement surgery, because she is still not a good surgical candidate. However, she has managed to get some of the insidious side effects of lack of mobility, such as weight gain and metabolic disease, under control.

Ms. G noticed increased tingling in her hands and arms. She loved to do arts and crafts, so this symptom became a significant source of angst for her. Nerve conduction studies showed she didn't have carpal tunnel syndrome, caused by ligamentous pressure on the median nerve to the middle fingers of the hand. Her problem originated in her cervical (neck) spine where the nerves to her arm and hand exited from the spinal cord through a bony vertebral opening. In her case, surgery was needed so she could get back to her hobbies. Of course, all of the nerves to our voluntary muscles have to come from the brain, and most traverse the spinal cord in their journeys. So, the spinal column can sometimes be the seat of musculoskeletal problems as it too ages.

All the above people had problems with their musculoskeletal systems, which interfered with their jobs, with mobility, and with living the lives they wanted to. Ultimately, if we live long enough, our bodies will get behind in the job of repairing microdamage and major insults. Wound healing is much slower the older we get.

The Lovely Bones: what the inside/structure of a bone looks like

When discussing the supporting structures of bones, knowing about the architecture of bones themselves becomes important. After all, bones have many tasks. They give structure to our bodies. Facial bones make us recognizable to others. Blood is manufactured in bones. Bones are a reservoir for minerals, especially calcium, which is essential for the function of all our cells. Of course, our bones are not developed fully when we are born. They need to grow and be assembled, or fused together, as we grow and go through adolescence. Let's look at a classical bone, called a long bone. The bones of your legs and arms are of this variety.

The epiphysis is the end of the bone. It is separated from the bone shaft or diaphysis by the metaphysis, a growth area. The bone marrow is present in some specific bones in adults, and is a red substance almost gelatinous in appearance, but very important. Tt is here that blood is produced.

Osteoporosis: fall and fracture prevention

Bones are an architectural wonder. Just like some public buildings, they are constantly undergoing remodeling, in response to the stresses of daily living. Let's say you take up running. Your leg bones will need to become stronger and perhaps to undergo some shape changing to accommodate the muscles and ligaments you are developing with your newfound activity. There are two main sets of cells charged with the duty of improving your tensile strength and bony architecture. The first of these cells is called an osteoblast, whose chore it is to create new bone. The osteoblast creates the matrix, or framework for bone, and lays down the calcium salts. The osteoclast, on the other hand, tears down bone which needs to be replaced. The process is analogous to dynamiting an old broken-down apartment on a city block to build a newer better structure (and in LA, one that is more earthquake proof)

Unfortunately, as people age, those osteoclasts do more tearing down than there are osteoblasts to rebuild the bone tissue. Loss of estrogen and diminution in testosterone levels doesn't help. For females, the years right after menopause herald a significant loss of bone. Once bone is thinner and has less structural strength, a condition called osteopenia or osteoporosis depending on severity, can cause a simple gravity fall to break a bone.

Mrs. H was a classic example. About a decade beyond menopause, she was walking her rather frisky dog and somehow became entangled in the leash, tripped and fell on her outstretched hands fracturing her right radius (one of two forearm bones, located on the thumb side of the forearm) This really put her out of commission because she was righthanded and had to be in a cast. That meant no cooking, no cleaning, no typing, it meant taking the bus wherever she needed to go, and it meant that she had to learn how to sleep differently, not tucked on her right side in fetal position. Getting dressed and other personal care issues became quite a challenge. Since she healed more slowly than an 18-year-old would, her cast began to seem like a permanent fixture.

The day the itchy, frayed cast was finally removed, Mrs. H had a question to which she demanded an answer. If her bones were so weak, how could she avoid another fracture, perhaps this time of her hip? Ms. H's mother had had a hip fracture, complicated by pneumonia, of which she had subsequently died. Of course that was several decades ago, and Ms H's mother was far older at the time, but the specter of her mother's long incapacitation, dependency and finally death haunted Ms. H.

A Dexa scan was ordered, a test to see if Ms. H's bones were osteoporotic. They were. Ms. H was Caucasian, and Caucasians and Asians have a higher risk of osteoporosis than persons of African descent, though family history is a game changer for everyone. Ms. H had fortunately given up smoking after her fracture, but alcohol consumption also could be an issue. Thyroid studies were done to rule out either a sluggish, or an overactive thyroid, both extremes causing bone problems. Ms. H's medications were given a thorough review, since some medications such as cortisol, are associated with structural wakening of bone. Ms. H was placed on daily vitamin D supplementation, calcium, and a regular exercise program. Osteoporosis can also be treated with medications, such as bisphosphonates and hormones, so an appropriate medication was also chosen specifically for Ms. H's needs. Lastly, Ms H's risk of falls was assessed. And the dog? She hired a neighbor teen to walk the beast.

The Joint: what makes joints hurt?

You have undoubtedly heard the term "snowbird" and may be aware that Florida has a population skewed towards seniors. Snowbirds are mature folk who spend winters in a warm climate, like Florida or Arizona, and summers in a more temperate climate, perhaps the Northeast. What is the reason for this unusual migration? Most seasonal migrants will blame their joints. But joints are not stand-alone structures and pain in the joints is generally tied to movement of said joints. Think about all the structures that make a joint work but that have pain fibers going to the brain via the spinal cord. These pain fibers can cause the perception of pain in the joint. Although cartilage covers the bones making up the joint, pain comes when cartilage is so worn away that the bony surfaces themselves are no longer protected. The synovial membrane makes the synovial fluid that lubricates the gliding motion of joints. Too much fluid because of joint pathology will cause pressure and pain, often described as "water on the knee". Ligaments give support to the bones of the joint but also limit joint motion. If a ligament is torn, the bones may move in ways they were not meant to, causing pain and collateral damage. Tendons and muscles move the bone that structurally ends as a component of the joint, to allow us to walk or throw a ball, for instance. Nerves in almost all these structures transmit pain messages to the brain: movement of a joint can uncover the structural problems that cause pain sensation in the brain. Changes of aging will undoubtedly cause some or all the joint structures to be damaged in some way. Interestingly, strengthening the muscles and tendons around a joint, ie keeping fit, reduces joint pain because muscles and their associated tendons can give the joint architectural support, much as using a cane would. Also, heat is a very good treatment for joint pain, increasing blood flow and allowing for local repair. It may be also that at a cellular level, warmth also permits optimization of metabolic reactions. As we age, our body temperature decreases. Babies are much warmer internally than grandmas, by a degree or two. If an 80 year old has a temperature of 99

Fahrenheit, which would be normal in an infant, most health providers look for infection. So it may be that the snowbird migration southward in cold weather is a population-based remedy for a phenomenon we haven't a complete grip on physiologically speaking. Of course, acute injuries respond to cold for a different reason, and that is to regulate the initial swelling.

Another difference between men and women: The aging of bones and joints

IF you want to avoid the leading cause of fractures in older Americans, which of course is osteoporosis, make sure that you are born an African male (or Japanese, or Native American… these will work too). Exercise every day or have a job for which regular exercise is a requirement. Keep on exercising after you retire. It helps to have a normal testosterone level into older age. Get lots of sun or take vitamin D daily if your level is below 30IU or so. Don't forget calcium, in your diet or by other means. Avoid thyroid malfunction, taking certain medications, smoking anything, and fast foods. Maintain a normal body weight and be careful about your alcohol intake.

Should you not care too much about bone health, be like Mrs. Q. She was new to the practice, of Caucasian ancestry, 65 years old, had an early menopause at 42 and smoked 2 packs a day. She also had a couple of beers almost every day. Her family history revealed that her mother had fractured a hip at age 69, never walked without assistance after that, and died the next year of pneumonia.

Mrs. Q's smoking habit had led to recurrent bouts of worsening asthma and chronic obstructive lung disease, for which she had received multiple courses of corticosteroids, medications known to cause bone loss but needed for her severe lung problems. Vegetables and meats were almost unheard of in her diet, since her husband had died, and she had no impetus to cook for herself. As for going outside in the sun, or exercising regularly, she counted walking upstairs several times a day to be sufficient. When she got the results of her bone density scan (DEXA), a test for bone health, she was horrified to learn of her osteoporosis diagnosis.

Women lose estrogen at the time of menopause, and this can be a rather abrupt loss. Men usually have a slower decline in testosterone levels. Both estrogens, from the ovaries, and testosterone, from the testes, support bone strength and health. This means men are generally at a lower risk for osteoporosis and the bone fractures it can lead to, than are women. Unfair, yes, but men can still get osteoporosis, especially when they get into their 70's and beyond. If you like to go online, google "FRAX" for a compilation of risk factors for osteoporosis which includes both men and women.

Day and night: What the time of day can tell you about causes of muscle, bone and joint pain

Mrs. A, a Spanish speaking woman in her mid-60's, came in complaining of knee pain. Accompanied by her daughter, she struggled to answer the triage nurse's very specific questions.

Both knees hurt, but the pain was diffuse. No, she couldn't put her finger on exactly where it hurt. With a sweeping gesture she emphasized that everything from mid shin to mid-thigh pained her. Which knee hurt more? Why both, of course. Her new physician, becoming more and more frustrated, finally turned to the daughter. It turned out that Mrs. A watched the daughter's three boys, aged 2months and 4 and 5 years, while the daughter was at work. Mrs. A's pain was worse in the evening, when she finally had a chance to sit down. Actually, sitting down wasn't the problem. It was getting up out of the chair after she had given herself a few moments to rest from the day's activities. And those stairs! Mrs. A had been running up and down three flights of stairs all day, so that by evening, she had to grip the banister and practically pull herself up. When she finally went to sleep, she had to avoid lying on her right side, because her right hip and posterior were very uncomfortable. X rays revealed osteoarthritis of the middle part of both knee joints, worse on the right, and arthritic changes in the right hip as well. An MRI of the right knee showed tears in her ligaments as well.

Mrs. B, on the other hand, was also in her md sixties. Her complaint was morning pain and stiffness in the shoulders and hips, which got better after an hour or so. She was not eating well, though she slept without discomfort, and her temperature hovered around 99 degrees, whereas normally it should have been about 97.5. Tests for rheumatoid arthritis, another disease that causes morning pain and stiffness were negative, but a test for inflammation, called the erythrocyte sedimentation rate, was wildly elevated.

Finding out what parts of the musculoskeletal system are causing trouble, and what to do about it, can be a real challenge in older folk, who can have more than one reason for pain in any given "geographic" area, and treatments can vary wildly as well. Some conditions are easily correctable. Others, often related to the aging process itself and the ability of an older person to undergo rigorous interventions like joint replacement, are not easily fixable. They demand either medical equipment like crutches or wheelchairs, or modification of the environment, like handrails or a home elevator.

Mrs. A responded to joint injections and modified babysitting but was told she would probably need a knee replacement in a few years. Mrs. B responded rapidly to a course of prednisone for her polymyalgia rheumatica. Another patient, Mrs. C, who had a stroke which left her with left sided muscle weakness allowing her to walk only a few steps at a time, needed a complete redo of her home after physical therapy failed to restore her to her former vigorous self. Her wheelchair was used for trips outside her home.

In general, a good history will include the daily peaks in musculoskeletal pain. Morning pain is more likely due to inflammatory processes like the synovial inflammation of joints. Pain towards evening may have its basis on stresses placed on aging joints by daily activities. Night pain of a particular anatomic area, let's say the shoulder, could point to tendons or ligaments previously damaged and tweaked by in inadvertent rolling over onto painful joint aggregates. Rarely in the young as well as their elders, an increase in night pain not associated with change in position may be associated with a more malignant diagnosis. When we are standing or even sitting, gravity adjusts body fluid downward. That is why people may often note more leg swelling from whatever cause as the day goes on. Conversely, when we lie flat at night, body fluid is more evenly distributed. (Remember, our bodies contain more water than anything) This can become a problem for people with heart failure, who must use pillows or sleep almost upright to keep their lungs from getting "boggy" with excess fluid. It can also either diminish or exacerbate pain elsewhere, particularly in the musculoskeletal system.

How people change their gait when bones, muscles, joints get "out of kilter"

Sometimes we can make diagnoses of bone and joint problems just by watching how people walk. Someone with a painful hip may have an antalgic gait. This means the person would bear weight on the painful leg for as short a time as possible.

A person who has weak hip abductor muscles (muscles found in the buttocks) will have drooping of the body to the side of these weak muscles.

Gait consists of two phases. During one phase, the foot is in contact with the ground, and this is called the stance phase. The swing phase is when the foot is in the air. If the foot and/or leg are weak, so that the foot can't clear the ground in the swing phase, a person will evidence circumlocution, The weak leg/foot will be swung outward in a semicircle to clear the ground instead of just swinging forward in a linear movement.

If a senior has a foot drop in which the foot cannot be flexed upward, that person will flex his or her hip and knee excessively to lift the foot, which may then flop down upon contact with the surface being walked on. This is called a foot slap.

Parkinsonism, depending upon its severity, can cause a whole host of walking problems. Festination is an unanticipated acceleration of gait, usually in the form of small steps. Freezing is just that. The person with Parkinsonism just stops moving at all for a short time. Propulsion is a falling forward and retropulsion a falling backward with ambulation.

Older folk naturally, without any specific neurologic pathology, will generally walk slower and swing their arms less as they walk. You may also have noticed, that because peripheral vision may diminish with age, people may walk in the center of a corridor or sidewalk, being unaware of faster walkers trying to pass them.

Many doctors will watch carefully as their patients walk to an exam room or attempt to get onto an exam table. Such observations can tell a lot about the state of the musculoskeletal system and of general health too.

One lady in her fifties, angling for state disability, had a decidedly antalgic gait (limp) as she ambled into the exam room, and evidenced great pain when asked to raise her arms above her head. Her doctor accidently dropped some change during the exam, at which point the patient swooped down to pick the money up. Another patient in her fifties had the stance of an eighty-year-old, walked trepidaceously, leaning on her cane. Her health care provider was about to sign a disability evaluation when a nurse rushed in. The erstwhile incapacitated lady, once out of the office, commenced to walk briskly swinging her cane in a circle above her head, and this behavior was observed by the passing nurse. Physicians in training, when evaluating younger patients for benefits, are advised to watch these patients as they go through the parking lot and/or get into their cars.

On the other hand, older people often put a lot of effort into walking correctly and can, when not tired or too stressed, appear to experience a better gait than they evidence routinely.

There is a brief test called the "get up and go" test, requiring a person to rise from a chair that has no arms, walk 6 feet, turn around and sit down in the chair again. A challenging test for persons with mobility problems, it can give information not only on gait but even on vision and equilibrium problems. Many older persons with gait issues will make heroic efforts, though, to complete this test normally! Some will not be able, due to balance or proprioception issues, to do the turn by using one foot and then the other in an arc-like maneuver. They will do a maneuver called "turning in bloc" wherein balance will not be shifted from one foot to the other but rather the whole body will be moved when executing a turn.

Environmental and activity changes to strengthen bones and joints and reduce pain.

When Mr. A, a freshly minted senior, came into the office for his routine diabetes check, he was wished a happy 65th birthday. His diabetes was under perfect control, as was his hypertension. In fact, it looked like some of his medications could be eliminated! AS he hopped up onto the exam table, he recalled with not a little pride, the efforts he had made to eat well and every day to walk at least 2 to 3 miles. As an additional benefit, he had discovered renewed energy and a marked decrease in the back pain that had plagued him since he had turned 60. In exercising daily, Mr. A had stumbled on the best medicine for bone and joint problems.

It is well known that hospitalized older patients lose muscle mass and musculoskeletal function very rapidly unless they are assisted to walk as soon as possible after admission. (8) (Kathleen T. Foley PhD OTR/L and Cynthia J. Brown, MD, MSPH, AGSF, in Chapter 20, Rehabilitation,, Geriatric Reviewe syllabus, 9th ed, Annette Medina-Walpole,MD, AGSF, et al,)

Mrs. T. who assented to a total hip replacement because just walking upstairs became a tortuous process, was "flabbergasted" when a physical therapist appeared at her bedside the day after her surgery. He proceeded to have her get up and take a step or two. Although Mrs. T wanted to vegetate after such a major operation, she was prodded and pushed to use her legs. To her amazement, she was out of the hospital and into rehab within five days. Soon the 66-year-old was going up and down stairs with the agility she had 10 years before.

Mrs H was a grandmother, a bit rotund, and at 59 was hardly geriatric. Unfortunately, in her culture, she was considered elderly and treated as such. She developed knee pain, which decreased her mobility, and this in turn increased her weight, which worsened her knee osteoarthritis. Her doctor explained to her that knee exercises, done daily, would strengthen the muscles supporting and moving her knees. This in turn would reduce her pain and stabilize her weight. Mrs. H would have none of it. Her passivity and attitude of resignation almost guaranteed that knee injections, physical therapy and non-narcotic pain killers would fail and she would graduate to a walker, playing out the role she believed her culture had predestined for her.

Bone and joint problems are such an expected issue as we age that preparing for them probably should start in middle age, if not before. Lifelong exercise increases muscle strength and joint mobility A good diet mitigates weight gain, which is a real problem especially for knees and hips. Folks who work using shoulders and arms repetitively may be at risk for shoulder rotator cuff damage. Don't forget mothers and fathers who routinely lift squirming, beefy toddlers and other things like grocery bags and furniture. Persons who have been athletes in high school, college and beyond, and who abruptly stop their sport, are at risk, and should plan on lifelong involvement in some sort of muscle activity, even if not their sport of choice.

How about if someone is already 65 and their knees and arms are giving trouble? Starting a graduated exercise program, perhaps with an 'exercise prescription" from one's health care provider, or even with specific recommendations from a physical therapist can work wonders. It is never too late to start moving joints and muscles, although the saying "start low and go slow" applies here as it does when new drugs are prescribed. Eating right helps too. Should finances and other commitments permit, a move to Florida or another Southern destination may be in the cards for Northerners. When a joint acts up, most geriatricians recommend staying away from that class of drugs called non-steroidal, and going instead to topical medications or appropriate doses of a medication like acetaminophen. Pain experts will caution to take medications regularly during a pain episode. If a medication is stopped when chronic pain is better, the pain will come back with a vengeance when the medication wears off. Bringing the pain level down will be more difficult than initially. Gait assistance devices like quad canes, and walkers may help during an acute bout of pain, with the objective of discontinuation after things simmer down. Wheelchairs can be a problem. Once in a wheelchair, it can be difficult to get back to ambulating. Eating one's regular diet will almost guarantee weight gain. People in wheelchairs use less energy, and need fewer calories, but such self control is difficult. The muscles and joints of the wheelchair- bound elderly quickly lose function. However, one intervention that really helps achy joints is the heating pad. Warmth applied to a troublesome back or shoulder can be the equivalent of a pain shot, without the side effects. Think about altering the environment when joint pain is inevitable.

How bones/joints/ligaments/bursae, vision/nerves and proprioception all work together to keep us upright.

You have probably been in a supermarket checkout line behind an elderly person who fidgets endlessly with a pack of bills before pulling out those required for payment. You tap your foot, and contemplate moving to another checkout line, but your items are already lined up on the checkout conveyer belt. Be aware that elderly person ahead of you is waging a mighty battle with waning proprioception, in this case involving the fine movements of the fingers and hand.

Our master computer, the brain, receives signals from the afferent nerves in joints, muscles, tendons and of course our sense organs such as the cochlea in the inner ear and the ophthalmic nerve in the eye. These "afferent" nerves sense position and movement changes through their respective structures and report these to the brain. The brain in turn amalgamates these incoming messages and sends out instructions to "efferent" nerves that tell muscles what to do. Unfortunately, nerves also age. They become less capable of growing new branches. The speed with which they transmit messages slows down. Muscle fibers lose some of the nerve connections that give them instructions from the brain.

But to keep upright, to be able to execute fine movements, to react to emergencies, both the nerves that give information to the brain and the nerves relaying instructions to the body from the brain have to be in working order. Nerves, however, can grow and resume lost function. It just takes a whole lot longer than it did when people were younger. Duplicated systems can often take over when one system fails. However, there is no substitute for keeping things in working order by using them.

The catastrophic effects of falls in the elderly: Hip fractures and their life altering effects

A slightly built lady in her seventies went shopping with a friend on a very windy day. She was in the process of opening the heavy door to a store, when a gust of wind blew the door towards her, and she fell, breaking her left hip. What followed was a trial pivoting this lady's will to regain independence against the effects of surgery, rehabilitation, and the real risk of depression and despair. The good news is that this woman won her half year battle to recuperate fully and was able to go back to the home where she had raised her children and resume independent living.

Many people are not so lucky. Although hips can fracture in different locations from the neck of the femur and relatively diagonally through the greater trochanter below the neck to rare fractures in the long part of the femur bone, most are related to osteoporosis. Many elderly people, who have osteoporosis and fracture a bone like the hip, also have other ailments that get worse during the recovery period from a fracture. Surgery, immobility, recuperation can all cause worsening of diabetes, can bring on lung problems, blood clots, muscle loss and even depression, among other complications.

In fact, having a hip fracture increases mortality by about 25% in the year following the fracture, and roughly1 in 4 persons will be in a nursing home a year after the fracture. Not good odds! (9) (Latham, NK, et al, Effect of a home-based exercise program on functional recovery following rehabilitation after hip fracture, JAMA. 2014;311 (7):700-708.

Wrist/forearm fractures and their effect on independence

She wasn't very sure of the type of fracture she'd had a year ago. It was her right wrist, she said. Her dog's leash had tripped her up, and she'd fallen on hands outstretched to brace herself. She was only 62, but had had an early menopause, a mother who'd died of a fractured hip, and a history of chain smoking.

By deduction, this lady probably sustained a Colles fracture. This type of fracture, though it can occur at any age, is common in an osteoporotic senior who has a fall from an upright position (gravity fall) onto outstretched hands and breaks the far end of the radius, one of the two forearm bones. The real problem come when the senior goes home in a cast and tries to do normal daily activities, especially if the dominant forearm/wrist was involved. Cooking, ironing, using a computer will all be challenges until that fracture heals. With a gravity fracture comes the need for treatment of osteoporosis. The person sustaining such a fracture. if the fracture didn't happen from falling from a height, implies weakened bones. The above patient was quickly placed on vitamin D and calcium after testing and invited to be on bone protective medications after a special bone study, called a DEXA scan, conclusively showed her osteoporosis.

Vertebral compression fractures are another type seen often in patients with loss of bone structure. They usually occur in the mid to lower back, and can be asympomatic or be a cause, to be differentiated from a host of other spinal conditions, of back pain. They can contribute to a humped back (kyphosis) and are sometimes hard to diagnose due to all the changes that take place in the spine over time. Keeping bones healthy and treating osteoporosis early can minimize these fractures as well.

Environmental detective work to avoid falls

The elder packrat

Her daughter was concerned that Mrs B was having an inordinate number of falls and near-falls. A home visit was called for. The pretty exterior of the Cape Cod home in a backstreet residential neighborhood belied the interior. Opening the front door was a problem. Piled high all over the living room and extending throughout the home were stacks of newspapers and magazines dating back perhaps 20-25 years. Clothing representing decades-ago fashions littered bedrooms. Knickknacks and souvenirs took up the remaining floor and shelf space. Anyone would fall in an environment like this.

Home obstacles can be a significant source of falls, and can range from wayward kittens to misplaced furniture. Excessive saving of mementos can indicate dementia or other psychologic ailments.

Steps, stairs and other obstacles

A home visit or a good environmental history can also reveal the steep stairs found in homes built over a century ago, or poor lighting, or perhaps unexpected step-downs between rooms . However, outside steps, often unrepaired after the altering effects of weather and usage, and stones and other obstacles like gopher holes in yards often cause more falls than indoor obstacles, with which an elderly person may be more familiar.

Seniors in an unfamiliar environment: when Grandma visits the grandkids

Navigating an unfamiliar environment requires use of all the senses, and a minimum of distraction. New places, particularly those not particularly senior friendly, can be a risk for falls.

How our clothes and shoes can hurt us

Imagine having restricted arm movement. How are you going to zip up a dress with a small back zipper? How about high heeled shoes, when you haven't worn them for months or years? What about seniors with reduced foot sensation, such as often affects folks with longstanding diabetes? Flip flops would certainly pose a risk for falls.

Mrs D encountered all of the above risk factors. She was visiting her rug-rat grandkids in another state, walking in bedroom slippers down a poorly lighted staircase in the early morning, and was distracted by thoughts of how she would spend the rest of the day. A slip and fall landed her on her posterior at the bottom of the staircase. Fortunately, there were only seven stairsteps, and she misplaced her foot on the third step, so there were no fractures, just a big bruise over her right gluteus (lower rear end)

Measures to prevent falls in seniors with specific medical issues (dropped foot, macular degeneration, etc) including social aspects: Obstacles and benefits

Seniors thrive as recognized members of a community, be it the family, a church group or an occupational setting. They also must shop and occasionally go to public places like restaurants, amusement parks or movies. AS our society grows more grey, public arenas will need to become more senior friendly, and seniors' function in these spaces optimized functionally. This is going to demand creativity on the part of everyone from architects and website designers to social workers, and rabbis, priests, ministers, imams!

What are the payoffs? Seniors will contribute more to society, and to their social circles. There will be less need for custodial senior care. Seniors will be happier, as will their families, and with healthier seniors, fewer funds will need to be diverted from other uses like education or road building. How about the obstacles? Our current world is designed for healthy young adults. Just look around at everything from subways to recreational equipment. WE are looking at a re-design of both public spaces and of living areas, of clothing, lighting, smart phones… you name it! Quite a challenge! Living through the Covid19 epidemic, though, has reinforced the need to keep seniors active and healthy, and of course out of assisted living where possible... This goal will take the combined efforts of middle aged people who are determined to live healthy lives in preparation for active golden years, older folk who recognize that they do have the power to improve their health and to make ongoing contributions to society, and a remodeling of the environment to anticipate the changes that take place in our bodies over time .

Seniors must do their part. This may mean deferring retirement, doing more babysitting, and most of all, staying healthy one's whole life so that there will be fewer health and motility problems as we age.

Finding the right exercise program to motivate

What about today's seniors? Disorders of muscles, joints and of motility in general often start in youth and are the principal reason for incapacitation. People set in their ways can be difficult to motivate. Work on many fronts needs to be done by both seniors and future seniors to change the culture and push, if necessary, those approaching or over 65 into living a healthy, vigorous and involved life where their productivity and effort counts.

CHAPTER 4

I can't pee/ hold my pee/get to the bathroom in time

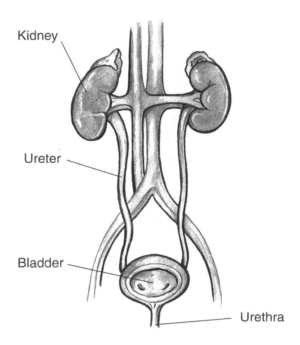

Kidney

Ureter

Bladder

Urethra

The female urogenital system: how it works

Mrs. T admitted reluctantly, while discussing her chronic insomnia, that she had to get up to urinate many times during the night. Recently, in an attempt to get to the bathroom quickly, she entangled her leg in the bedding, almost falling on her face. In the process of recovering balance, she had urinated quite a bit. She was now very sensitive to how much fluid she drank before bedtime, and had trained herself to become a light sleeper, even considering setting her alarm to awaken and evacuate her bladder before her bladder awakened her. The latter plan had to be abandoned since the alarm would also awaken her husband. It seemed that this anxiety about urinating may be playing a role in her sleeping difficulties.

The urinary tract, composed of kidneys, ureters, bladder and urethra, is a remarkable model of engineering. Let's take the kidney, male or female, first. The kidney's mission is to remove toxic and waste material from the blood stream. (The liver plays a role independent of the kidneys in neutralizing or eliminating waste and toxins)

The kidneys sit in the upper back of the abdomen. Their location is the reason that people with kidney infections (pyelonephritis) or kidney stones (nephrolithiasis) often feel pain in their midbacks. The kidneys are shaped like rather big (10 cm or so) kidney beans, the latter being so named for obvious reasons. They have an elaborate method for filtering waste and retrieving important substances after filtration. They also help balance the pH of our blood when instructed to do so by hormones/nerves etc.

The renal artery sends blood to the kidneys, and the arterial blood vessels divide progressively, finally becoming small "afferent" arterioles. These blood vessels then form a tuft of smaller blood vessels or capillaries within the glomerulus, a structure surrounded by a capsule known as Bowman's Capsule where filtered waste products from the blood now enter the nephron as the beginnings of urine formation. The cleansed blood meanwhile exits the glomerulus and goes back to the circulation, newly waste-free, through the so-called "efferent" arterioles. The waste products, known as urine, then traverse the rest of the nephron downstream of Bowman's capsule, which is the structure mentioned above at which the initial filtration has taken place. The nephron, a convoluted tubule where each portion accomplishes separate tasks of filtration, regulates the pH or acidity/alkalinity of the body through adding or subtracting molecules like sodium and calcium from the urine. Each segment of the nephron has its own duties and responds to orders from hormones, chemicals and the nervous system. For example a hormone called antidiuretic hormone, made in the hypothalamus of the brain and released by the pituitary gland, when it is alerted by specific parts of the nervous system or by other hormones, tells the nephron that the body is getting dehydrated, so specific parts of the nephron are instructed to squeeze more water out of the urine and return it to the body. Doing so will make the urine more concentrated, and the urine will look darker than usual. Most of us are endowed with about a million nephrons in our prime.

Ok, the kidney with its flagship structure, the nephron, has filtered and processed the urine, preserving electrolyte balance and hydration in the body itself, and ridding the body of waste and toxins. Now the urine travels down the ureter, a tube that connects the kidneys with the bladder. When the bladder gets close to filling, neurons (nerves) in the bladder alert the brain, and the urge to void begins. Waves of bladder contractions get more insistent that we find an appropriate place to void. Voiding, or "emptying the bladder", takes place through another tube called the urethra. Meanwhile a valve where the bladder connects with the urethra, called the internal urethral sphincter, holds tight, while another valve, called the external urethral sphincter, this one under our voluntary control, also closes against the ever increasing urge to void. In Mrs. T's case, a couple of things went array, leading to complications like a near fall and even trouble sleeping

Effects of pregnancies on bladder function and the ability to hold urine

Anatomically, women have an area called the vulva, between the legs and composed of two diverging ridges of tissue called the labia or lips, at whose apex is the clitoris. Within the labia, three important organs terminate or end. These organ systems include the bladder, the uterus/ vagina with its associated ovaries and tubes, and the rectum, which is the last segment of the colon. All reside in a bowl like area called the pelvis, situated below the abdomen and contained within the confines of the pelvic bones. The first organ opening, nearest the clitoris, is the urethra, carrying urine from the bladder. The second tube or opening is the vagina, partially covered by a membrane called the hymen. The hymen is the membrane subject to inspection in the olden days and even now in certain cultures, to see if a girl is still a virgin. It generally is ruptured with first intercourse, leading to slight bleeding when a young woman initially has sex. However, we now know that the hymen may be opened due to ordinary childhood activities or minor injuries, or may be thin and incomplete, so its presence or absence is not really a test of virginity as was believed in days of yore.

The third opening, usually a bit behind the other two, is of course the rectum, at the end of the large bowel or colon, where stool is evacuated.

When a woman is carrying a growing baby in her uterus, downward forces may stretch the ligaments and muscles which make up the pelvic floor, and which, more importantly, hold the bladder, uterus, and rectum in place. This stretching may ultimately cause the bladder and even the uterus to shift position or the walls of the rectum or bladder to balloon out, weakening the valves that hold urine in the bladder to prevent untimely voiding. AS women age` this weakening of the "suspensory ligaments", so called because they keep the organs of the pelvis in place like the suspensory cables of a bridge, start to weaken. As this happens, the organs of the pelvis can "prolapse" or sink downward. When these organs are displaced from their pristine positions, they cannot do their job well. Women will complain of loss of urine at inappropriate times (urge incontinence), or when they cough (stress incontinence) or of a backup of urine when the bladder isn't emptying completely. Additional problems include the uterus dropping downward, or a ballooning out of the weakened walls of either the urethra (urethrocele) or the rectum (rectocele).

Poor Mrs. A was severely demented. She had lived a good life, given birth to several children, but her Alzheimer's disease eventually landed her in a nursing home. However, her daughter was still very much involved in her care and brought her to see her doctor for a pelvic exam and pap smear. To everyone's surprise, and to the chagrin of the nursing home staff, a problem with Mrs. A's uterus was discovered for the first time. The mouth of the uterus (cervix) was hanging out of the vagina and dragging the uterus itself downward. Only Mrs. A's dubious mental status had kept her from articulating her discomfort.

Many perfectly normal women suffer from so-called "key in the door" or urge incontinence. Like Mrs. B She had a baker's half dozen of kids, all happily grown, married, employed. What started as a rare event when her bladder was quite full had evolved into an almost everyday occurrence. When she got home from work or shopping, and knew she needed to void, the minute she parked and exited her car, she would involuntarily leak. It wasn't very much, and sometimes if she anticipated the problem and clamped down really hard, it wouldn't happen. However, she had altered her routine sufficiently to forestall the event by locating all the bathrooms everywhere she went and being sure to use them before heading back home.

Had she discussed this problem with her doctor, she would have become aware that urge incontinence can often be treated quite successfully with medication. Mrs. B, however, was too embarrassed to broach the subject with her best friend, let alone a physician.

Mrs. C's loss of urine happened when she tried to jump on her son's trampoline. She gave up jumping. Then it happened again when she had a bad cold. Every paroxysm of coughing would be followed by a tiny accident. Pretty soon she was worried about incontinence when she had a giggle fit. Mrs. C's problem was a bit less amenable to correction. She would probably need a surgical procedure for her stress incontinence, which occurred whenever she experienced increased abdominal pressure. Meanwhile she wore pads everywhere....so she could cough, or laugh should the occasion arise.

Some women have more than one kind of urine loss, so a thorough evaluation for such conditions as bladder infection or rarely a mass or neurologic problem needs to happen before a decision can be made about treatment.

Social effects of incontinence: embarrassment and withdrawal

Although many women, even those who haven't had a pregnancy, eventually have some form of urinary incontinence, it is not considered a socially acceptable topic. Since significant incontinence makes itself known, many women resort to wearing extra strength menstrual pads, refraining from sports, scouting out bathrooms wherever they go, or not drinking needed fluids. Some may even become reclusive. For others, adult diapers have been a lifesaver. In the long run, this taboo topic needs to be considered more openly because a lot of people continue to suffer in silence!

Changes in sexual function after menopause and how they affect quality of life (or not!)

Perimenopause is that sometimes prolonged period in a woman's life when her ovaries sputter and sometimes fail to produce enough hormone to induce regular menses or periods. The ovaries have a limited number of oocytes…cells which will grow and become ova, be released by the ovary and when fertilized, travel to the uterus, snuggle in its cushy lining, absorbing nutrition through the developing placenta and umbilical cord and emerge as an amazing newborn. The ovaries also produce estrogen and progesterone. Estrogen is produced alone by the ovaries until a woman's midcycle, usually halfway between two menses. Then the brain's hypothalamus, which acts as the ovary's "boss", secreting messenger hormones to direct what the ovary should be doing, sends a powerful hormonal signal. This signal in the form of the hormone LH or luteinizing hormone, tells the ovary to release the oocyte which has now matured into an ovum, for its travel down the fallopian tube to be fertilized by the male's sperm. Meanwhile the ovary now also produces a hormone called progesterone which prepares the endometrium, the lining of the uterus mentioned above, to receive the fertilized egg with its now complete genetic instructions on how to develop into a mature baby. Generally during the fertile period of a woman's life, this cycle repeats itself every month. If the released egg is not fertilized, the uterus sheds its prepared lining in the form of menstrual flow or "blood" and the cycle repeats itself the next month.

Finally, a woman runs out of oocytes, and she enters menopause, and can't get pregnant anymore. Most women become menopausal at about age 51, but there is a lot of variation. The ovaries shrivel and cease to produce much hormone. When this happens, all the great benefits those hormones confer on females also decline. Estrogens (and progesterone in part) have functions in every organ from the skin and bladder through to the bones. About 80% of women will also have "hot flashes" as their bodies complain about the loss of female hormones. These hot flashes are comprised of a feeling of a heat wave involving the upper part of the body, followed by sweating which can be rather drenching. They can continue for months to years and even decades, and can interfere with sleep, making not a few women grumpy and irritable. Eventually they disappear.

One duty of estrogens is to lubricate the vagina, so intercourse often can become unpleasant when estrogen production diminishes. Many women will feel unattractive, some even depressed, and a few will experience enough discomfort to try and avoid intercourse (sex). The "change of life" can also bring less pleasure with sex, and this can be quite upsetting to women who have had a great sex life.

On the other hand, many women are happy to be relieved of the risk of an inadvertent pregnancy, although perimenopausal pregnancies, occurring when the ovaries are still in a sputtering stage, have been known to occur. My favorite story involved a fifty-one-year-old woman who had married in her teens, had 10 or 11 children, raised them all, and then discovered herself pregnant at age fifty. She gave birth to a perfect baby girl. However, she had long ago diapered and nursed her last infant and was as worried as a first time mom about caring for this new arrival. Her grown daughters, all with children of their own, took turns on coming to visit the new mom and helping her raise this unexpected (but cherished) baby.

My most frustrating tale was that of the elegant menopausal lady who was extremely angry at me and at medicine in general. She was furious that we couldn't resurrect her aging ovaries and give her the sexual pleasure she'd enjoyed in her younger days. However, her problem was broader than just the loss of youthful hormones. She was depressed. The disease of depression can cause a lack of libido in even a well-endowed, hormone-rich thirty-year-old. Sometimes working with factors other than a lack of hormones can resurrect a love life gone south, and this may include everything from looking at optimizing sexual techniques to spending time with one's spouse away from the responsibilities and worries of ordinary life, even if only for an occasional evening. A mature love life can be satisfying in a way different from, but as wonderful in its own way, as the exciting love life of youth. Most couples will find their own paths through this uncharted territory.

Ways of identifying and dealing with common urogenital problems

Although hormones help with issues like hot flashes and bone loss, not even the addition of the male hormone testosterone can fully reverse the changes aging wrecks on the female genital apparatus. All hormonal treatment has both benefits and drawbacks, and the use of hormones is a very individual decision made with full understanding of known risks and benefits and also with a knowledge of family genetics.

Incontinence of course is a mixed bag. A thorough history and physical exam, including a pelvic exam, and testing needs to be done to identify exactly where and what is the probable cause. Prolapsed or "fallen" organs can be treated mechanically, with a device called a pessary, to push up and support a displaced uterus. Some lucky and persistent women who have only stress incontinence can even exercise their pelvic muscles to the point where they keep organs in place....somewhat like training for a marathon. Usually, a physical therapist, trained in female incontinence problems, becomes a coach. She can teach exercises like the well-known Kegel's and with diligence make a real difference in continence care .

The male urogenital system: how it works

Men's kidneys, ureters and bladders work pretty much the same as women's. However, the male urethra is surrounded by the prostate, an organ which has an important reproductive function. Sperm made in the testes travel to the prostate, an organ that produces a slightly alkaline fluid which is propelled by the muscular part of the prostate along with the sperm into the urethra and then out the penis with ejaculation (orgasm, coming).

The growing prostate and the problems it can cause

This organ starts out about the size of a walnut but grows in most men throughout life and can choke the urethra as it carries urine from the bladder to the outside. When this happens, the urine can back up and cause damage to all the structures upstream including the bladder, ureters, and kidneys. (10) (Anatomy of the prostate gland, Johns Hopkins Medicine.org, health library)

Mr. T was really in distress. Initially his symptoms included having to get up often at night to urinate, aggravated by an infuriatingly slow stream, and dribbling of urine. He had seen his urologist and had been placed on medications for his big prostate. Things went along ok for a while, but then one day he couldn't pee much at all. His urologist inserted a catheter into his bladder to drain the urine that was being blocked, but when it was taken out, the problem happened all over again. It happened on a weekend, when his urologist was off call, necessitating a visit to urgent care. Once again, in went the catheter, not a pleasant procedure, a culture was done for infection, and Mr. T was referred to his urologist for further expert treatment. Most men, fortunately, don't have a prostate that grows to the point of choking off urethral urine flow, but most men who live into old age will have prostates that grow to the point where they cause some voiding problems.

Mr Z was even unluckier. His prostate had grown, and he had ignored distant early warning symptoms. Eventually urine, which couldn't get out easily through his very squeezed urethra, built up in the bladder, reaching to the kidneys. Finally, very little urine was expelled, and Mr. Z needed an operation…urgently…lest his kidneys be permanently injured from the backed-up pressure of his urine.

Of course, hiding behind an enlarged prostate is always the prospect of a hidden cancer. Many prostate cancers are very slow growing, small and never cause problems. A few are vicious, growing fast and spreading to the bones and other organs. Prostate cancer also seems to run in families, and for unknown reasons, African Americans are more at risk than others. Therefore, a urologist will generally check carefully for an unidentified cancer lurking in a big prostate, especially one with suspicious nodular areas.

Erectile Dysfunction, lots of problems, only a few remedies

Mr. W was clearly mandated to see a doctor by his wife. However, he didn't get down to business till the very end of his appointment. First, he talked about his sniffles, then a minor rash. Finally, it came out. "Hey Doc, I'm having this trouble…." His physician knew before the sentence was finished what the problem was. Most men, especially as they get older, will suffer occasionally or even all the time from ED and other common sexually related problems including low desire and abnormal ejaculation. These are difficult topics to discuss, for many reasons. Health care professionals want to help, and generally have had lots of experience discussing the issue with lots of different men. First, an overview. Loss of libido, or interest in sex, can stem from many causes, including the medicines or even recreational drugs a man is taking, depression, other illness he may have, using pornography, and sometimes his relationship with his sexual partner.

One gentleman, only in his late thirties, came in complaining of inability to get an erection with his wife. Further questioning revealed that he performed well with his mistress. A year passed and he was back again. Same problem. This time, he could perform neither with his wife, nor with his initial mistress. However, he was performing just fine with his new mistress. It was suggested that he see a psychiatrist......or a priest or minister!

However, ED itself can take several forms. Premature ejaculation refers to when a man "comes" too soon, within 1 minute of vaginal penetration. Retrograde ejaculation can happen in certain diseases like diabetes, or rarely with specific medications, or if the neck of the bladder is damaged and can't close as sometimes happens after prostate surgery. Failure to ejaculate can happen with medications like Tamsulosin, used itself to help men with enlarging prostates, and with certain medications used for depression.

Evaluation of ED consists of having a thorough history and physical exam looking for diseases, medicines, psychologic issues and surgical procedures which may be causative, doing laboratory testing for hormones from the brain and the testes (balls) and then introducing treatments appropriate for the condition or conditions causing ED. Men have to know that their problem is neither unique nor embarrassing, and deserves the evaluation and treatment that any medical issue should be accorded. (11) ("Evaluation of male sexual dysfunction", Glenn R. Cunningham, MD, Mohit M. Khera, MD. MBA. MHP in Up To Date, section Editor, Peter J. Snyder, MD, Alvin M. Matsumoto, MD, Michael P. O'Leary, MD, MPH)

Common kidney and bladder problems that affect both men and women: Kidney stones

Mrs T awoke with severe colicky pain coming from her left flank and traveling to the left abdomen. She recognized immediately, and with some chagrin, what was happening. It had happened before. Mrs T had another kidney stone, and it was traveling down her ureter and, in the process, giving her as much pain as when she had given birth to her daughter. She was a stone former and had become very lax about drinking lots of water to avoid stone formation in her kidney.

Most of us remember high school science projects, where we mixed salt or perhaps sugar in warm water, creating a supersaturated solution. As the water cooled and evaporated, crystals would form. Unfortunately, this process can also happen in some folks' kidneys, creating kidney stones which can pass down the ureters, into the bladder, and be passed, with luck, through the urethra and eliminated. If the stone being passed is big, it can cause a lot of pain, bleeding into the urine and even infection.

Urinary infections and other issues, including indwelling catheters

Mrs. Q was a grandmother with a fever. When her grandson stopped by to deliver her weekly groceries, he could tell something was very wrong. Mrs. Q, a sprightly widow in her late seventies, usually kidded him about his girlfriend and his "souped up" car. Today she seemed listless, and her conversation disjointed and sparse. He called his mother and soon Mrs. Q was in the emergency room being admitted to the hospital. She had a condition called urosepsis, meaning that a bad kidney infection was leaking bacteria into her bloodstream. Her urine was cultured to identify bacteria and target the infection with the correct antibiotic, and she was immediately started on an antibiotic likely to kill the types of bacteria most likely to be causing the trouble. Luckily, she responded well, her fever, rapid pulse and shaky blood pressure normalizing, and her confused thinking becoming more rational.

The urinary tract can be a site of serious infection in older folk. Many seniors, perhaps 1 in 5 women and 1 in ten men have bacteria in their urine, that aren't causing any harm. However, bacteria in the bladder that are causing symptoms need to be treated, usually with antibiotics. These worrisome symptoms can range from burning when urinating, to going with increased frequency and urinating small amounts very frequently, to causing or worsening of incontinence or involuntary loss of urine. Sometimes the kidneys can become infected, and here we get into more serious territory, because seniors with kidney infections can have fever, back pain, and are at risk for urosepsis, the condition Mrs. Q had. This is a medical emergency, needing urgent antibiotic treatment. Some older individuals with urosepsis will present in unusual ways, for example, becoming confused and listless, and having low blood pressure and a rapid heart rate, and sometimes even becoming hypothermic (having a body temperature much lower than normal).

Men can also suffer from prostate, testicular and epididymal pain, swelling or tenderness, with pain seeming to track to the scrotum in some infections. (12) (Manisha Juthani-Mehta, MD and Theresa A. Rowe, DO, Chapter 62, Infectious Diseases, in Geriatric Review Syllibus, 9th edition, American Geriatrics Society, Annette Medina-Walpole. MD, AGSF, James T.Pacala, MD, MS, AGSF, and Jane F. Potter, MD, AGSF Editors in Chief)

Kidney failure

Mr. F had had diabetes for at least two decades, and unfortunately, when he first developed this very common genetic metabolic disease, was cavalier about following a good diet and taking his medications regularly. Now he was in his mid-sixties, and his doctor told him that his kidneys were failing, couldn't filter the waste out of his body properly, and that he would need dialysis soon. Dialysis is a process where the blood is cleansed of waste through a machine, and patients generally go to a nearby dialysis center and are hooked up to the machine for several hours about three times a week for this process. In order to cleanse the blood, a shunt between an artery and vein must be surgically created, usually in the arm. This is where the attachment to the dialysis machine takes place. Shunts are generally created months before absolute kidney failure is expected to take place, so that they will be ready or mature when needed. Sometimes, if kidneys fail very rapidly because of a bad disease process, emergency dialysis has to occur till the disease is better. Another form of dialysis is called peritoneal dialysis, and this form uses the placement of special fluid in the abdomen to which waste will be transferred through peritoneal or abdominal membranes, and then the removal of the now waste-laden fluid, on a regular basis.

Fortunately, there are grades of kidney failure, and most persons don't reach the degree of failure where dialysis is necessary. In fact, most seniors do experience a mild degree of kidney failure that waxes and wanes, and slows down the process of waste elimination a bit, but is clinically pretty inconsequential. This is because as we age, our kidneys change, lose nephrons, and glomeruli and are just not quite as efficient as they were in youth.

Dementia and Incontinence

When we think of incontinence, involuntary loss of urine (or sometimes stool or both) due to medications, injuries or physiologic changes of aging comes to mind. However, not getting to the toilet in a timely manner can also be a factor in incontinence. So can failure to recognize bodily clues telling of the need to void! Persons with developmental delay from birth and persons with dementia may have done well earlier in life, but the changes of aging added to the changes of their diseases ay push them over the edge. As we age, bladder contractions become more variable and may decrease or become hard to control, urine output can be shifted to later in the day, the bladder has a smaller reservoir for holding urine, and of course, medication use generally increases as we age. Lots of different medications can interfere with the entire process of voiding. For example, persons on diuretics, which are medications to remove excess water from the body and to control blood pressure, will accumulate urine and must void more often when the medication works.

Now imagine someone who has problems walking, or getting out of bed, or can't see very well in the dark. Add to this a problem remembering how to get to the bathroom and what to do upon getting there. You can see that even mild dementia can lead to urinating (or defecating) in the wrong place, or perhaps before getting to the toilet, removing clothes appropriately and sitting down in the right place. But demented persons may also have other forms of incontinence, and these too must be addressed A good history and physical must be done to the extent possible to correct whatever internal problems, medications, and external factors may be contributing to inappropriate loss of urine (or stool).

Daycare programs for persons with disabilities and dementia often use special strategies like timed voiding before accidents can occur, and also of communicating with the demented person on a level he or she can understand to get into a pattern of voiding appropriately. This communication can sometimes take the form of telling a senior with toileting forgetfulness that it is time for a walk. The walk leads to the bathroom, and often the senior, seeing the bathroom, will suddenly remember that she does need to use the facilities!

Identification of incontinence in men and women: medical behavioral and device treatments

Consider the sad story of Mr. F, made more tragic because after a couple of visits to his health care provider, he disappeared. Mr. F, as is the case with so many other older folk, led a lonely life. He lived by himself in a rented room in the big city. He had lost the love of his life many years ago, why and how he would never reveal. When he was first seen, it was obvious that incontinence was one of his problems. His ill-fitting baggy pants had a ring of self-evident moisture in the front of the crotch. He apparently was unaware of his dribbling. However, other issues were so pressing that incontinence was put on the back burner. After his second visit, he never returned and attempts to reach him were futile.

Although most persons with incontinence are not as elusive as poor Mr. F, there is a significant social stigma to incontinence. People do not want to reveal their symptoms to their health care providers, so nurses, doctors, physicians' assistants, medical assistants, nurse practitioners…. all of us…. must go out of our way to ask about such problems. Then we must ask about the circumstances under which loss of urine occurs. Does it happen when a person is laughing, or running, or coughing? All these activities increase intraabdominal pressure which can cause stress incontinence leakage. Does coming home and knowing that a bathroom is nearby trigger the brain to call for premature expulsion of urine before the toilet is reached? Urge incontinence may be the culprit. Has the patient damaged his spine, where the nerves of urination (and defecation) hang out? Does the patient have arthritis or other musculoskeletal issues that make getting out of bed at night to urinate a difficult, painful and slow process? Is the patient always thirsty and drinking a lot of water? More than one case of diabetes has been diagnosed based on a history of this type of incontinence. Or perhaps a good history reveals symptoms of a bladder infection, or of more than one of the conditions leading to involuntary loss of urine (mixed incontinence). Check medications.

Next comes the physical exam. A thorough pelvic exam may reveal a prolapse (descent of a structure that is not held properly in place due to weakening of muscles and ligaments in the pelvis). The rectal exam may show a big prostate in an older man. A neurologic exam may reveal numbness associated with the nerves which control voiding. Maybe imaging studies, like an ultrasound will show something in the area which needs to be corrected. Once there is a preliminary identification of what the patient's problem could be, medications or even surgery may be called for, and referral to an appropriate specialist provided.

The most important part of identification of incontinence in either a man or a woman is getting him or her to tell the provider that a problem in this sphere exists!

CHAPTER 5

The "Ticker" and Its Connections: with some notes on how you got a heart

There is a remarkable story behind how you acquired your heart. Long, long ago, one cell creatures came into existence. Their basic needs were pretty much the same as those of an elephant, a shark, or tyrannosaurus rex…or you and I. They had to catch food, take it into their little bodies, break it down and distribute the "fragments" within their simple bodily structures. They also had to grab onto some oxygen for respiration. Finally, they had to get rid of the accumulated waste products from their metabolism. These steps were accomplished through diffusion through cell membranes. Now diffusion through a membrane is fine if you are a one celled creature. It is a slow process, but it works.

However. If your body is composed of billions of oxygen-and-food hungry cells, you need a more sophisticated method of getting your metabolic needs met. Insects and crustaceans devised an "open" circulatory system where their blood, called hemolymph, bathed their organs. Vertebrates needed something even more sophisticated, a closed vascular system consisting of a complex network of tubes or blood vessels lined with specialized epithelial cells. And the oxygen wasn't just dissolved in hemolymph. It was packaged in neat, biconcave disc-like contraptions we call red blood cells, attached to specialized structures called hemoglobin. Of course, something is needed to propel the fluid within those tubes or blood vessels, and that something is a pump called the heart. Most vertebrates also have another system, called the lymphatic system, which brings interstitial fluid- the fluid between our cells- back to the circulation. More about how these systems hook up later!

Now about the heart. If you were a fish, your heart would have an atrium, where the blood from the body in need of reoxygenation collects, and a ventricle, the pumping chamber in series with the oxygen exchanging gills, where the blood is again resupplied with the oxygen dissolved in water, thence to be transported to all fishy cells and organs.(13) (Evolutionary origins of the blood vascular system and endothelium, r. Monahan-Earley, A,M, Dvorak, W.C. Aird, Journal of Thrombosis and Haemostasis, Vol. 11, issue 51)

The basic structure of the heart and circulatory system

The human oxygen and food delivery system is much more complex, and its complexity both allows us to function and also sets us up for problems like atherosclerosis (hardening of the arteries) and pulmonary emboli (blood clots within the big pulmonary vessels bringing blood to the lungs to get more oxygen).

First the heart, which according to Web MD is a fascinating muscle. It pumps 2000 gallons of blood a day through 60,000 miles of blood vessels. That is roughly the equivalent in mileage of going back and forth across the US ten times! Our hearts have four chambers. The right atrium receives blood loaded with the waste product carbon dioxide and collected from all the body's cells. This returning blood has given up its oxygen to all those bodily cells, received carbon dioxide in return, and will return the carbon dioxide to the lungs to be gotten rid of as we exhale. The right ventricle is a pumping chamber. The blood from the right atrium passes through a valve called the tricuspid, which then closes as the right ventricle contracts, propelling the blood through the pulmonary valve into the pulmonary artery and thence to a web of smaller vessels called arterioles, and finally to the capillaries of the lungs where the actual freshening of the blood with newly inhaled oxygen occurs via very small capillary lined structures called alveoli. Carbon dioxide goes into the alveoli during this process and is exhaled via bronchi and trachea, and lovingly received by green trees and plants in their metabolic processes.

Back to the newly oxygenated blood. It then returns by way of the pulmonary veins to the left atrium, splashes through the mitral valve to the left ventricle, another more powerful pumping chamber, which shoves the now oxygen-rich blood through the aorta. Since all four chambers of the heart are in some way employed in the main function of the heart, which of course is propelling blood all around the body, how does the heart get its instructions on the timing and force of its pumping activity? Actually, the heart, besides being a powerful muscle, is also an electrical system.

A quick overview of the heart's electrical system and pumping function

The electrical system of the heart is composed of specialized muscle cells capable of generating electrical impulses, as are all heart muscle cells to some degree. The electrical impulses start at the sinoatrial node, located high up in the right atrium. This collection of specialized cells produces an electrical impulse called an action potential, which travels down to the atrioventricular node and starts a sequential contraction of the chambers of the heart. These generated contractions of the heart muscles are what pumps the blood. The atrioventricular node, located near the coronary sinus, receives the electrical impulses from the sinoatrial node and spreads these impulses to the muscles of the ventricles, again by way of a specialized network of Purkinje cells causing these powerful pumping chambers to contract, sending blood to the lungs (right ventricle) or to the body through the aorta. Through this electronic network, the atria receive the signal to contract first, sending blood to the ventricles. When the ventricles are filled with the blood from the atria, they are then told to contract. You can see that this is an exquisitely timed system allowing the upper and lower chambers of the heart to fill with and then empty blood in a way that optimizes the pumping function of the heart. It is further influenced by hormones and other input which signals the heart's conducting system to force a more rapid, or a slower, rate of pumping.

Mr. Lopez was only 63, but he hadn't worked for years. His hypertension brought him into the clinic, but he also had a complaint about his energy level. It was true that Mr. Lopez's life was quite low key. He would get up around 9 or 10 am, amble over to the local donut shop for a breakfast of jelly donuts, orange juice and coffee, grouse about life with his buddies who also frequented the donut shop, walk a half block home, settle down to a TV show during which he usually fell asleep, awake for his TV dinner, you get the picture. His complaint about easy fatigability caught his physician by surprise until the doctor did a heart exam. Mr. Lopez's heart rate was somewhat erratic. An electrocardiogram demonstrated a flaw in his cardiac conduction system called atria fibrillation. In this condition, the upper chambers or atria of the heartbeat in a disorganized fashion so the atria do not send specific aliquots of blood to the ventricles in a regular fashion to be pumped out. Of course, Mr. Lopez was fatigued! This condition is more likely to occur the older we get and can be quite subtle. It is treatable, and Mr. Lopez soon had enough energy to pursue his regular daily activities. Like other heart and circulatory problems, symptoms can be abrupt or sneaky, and may be masked and evidenced only by a decline in a person's usual activity.

The heart, being a big muscle, which starts its lifelong work when we have been in our mother's womb for about 4 weeks, needs a hearty, constant source of blood delivery and the ability to step up flow at a second's notice. The coronary arteries, which come off of the aorta (see below) almost immediately, supply that need. In most folk, the left coronary artery, which splits into the left anterior descending and circumflex arteries, feeds the left atrium, ventricle and interventricular septum. The right coronary artery gives nourishment and oxygen to the heart conduction system, right atrium and parts of the ventricles. These blood vessels are very important, because blockage causes a heart attack, and the muscle cells in the portions of the heart watered by the obstructed blood vessel will die. Again, atherosclerotic blockage and rupture is more common as we age. However, there are anomalies of the coronary blood vessels in many people, mostly benign. Rare anomalies can cause a heart attack sooner.

A very astute pediatrician sent a year-old boy by helicopter transfer from a small city with few pediatric specialists to a big city children's hospital with the diagnosis of myocardial infarction or heart attack. This little fellow was short of breath, fatigued and growing slowly. Things became critical, and an EKG, which tells what coronary blood vessels may not be working by way of an assessment of the conduction system of the heart, was abnormal. The pediatrician, after seeing the electrocardiogram or EKG, quickly surmised that the tyke had an improperly formed coronary artery, and parts of the heart muscle were being deprived of blood. This pediatrician acted with lightning speed to get a pediatric heart surgeon to see and operate on the infant and saved the child's life.

The above situation is very unusual, because the reason for most heart attacks most often has to do with slowly acting genetic factors, with poor lifestyle practices, and with the effects of aging.

Arteries, arterioles and capillaries: the body's freeway system

Back to the aorta, a big artery which distributes the blood to successively smaller blood vessels, the branch arteries, arterioles, and finally capillaries. Capillaries are extremely small blood vessels which are intimate with all the cells of the body and where the true work of oxygen exchange and carbon dioxide elimination takes place. The arteries of the head and upper extremities branch first from the aorta. The brain especially has a high metabolic rate, demanding a fairly large supply of nourishment and oxygen through the brachiocephalic, left common carotid and left subclavian arteries. Since humans (and all other living creatures) need more than oxygen (or carbon dioxide if you are a green plant) to survive, the next group of arterial branches from the mighty aorta feed the digestive system. These arteries are the superior mesenteric and the hepatic arteries. And the renal arteries feed the kidneys, where waste is eliminated in the form of urine. The common iliac arteries bifurcate or split from the aorta and feed the legs . There are other branches from the aorta, and from the iliac arteries. that supply the bowel, and genital organs with blood. Successive branching of these more major arteries to smaller and smaller arterioles finally leads to the above mentioned capillary beds where the true work of supplying individual cells with energy and oxygen, and of removing waste actually takes place, just as it would in a one cell creature interfacing with the watery environment to provide these services.

Veins and venules: the way back to the heart

After the body's cells get their needs met for food and oxygen through their interface with those very tiny capillaries, the now deoxygenated blood, having had its nutritional load given up to the cells, has to get back to the right side of the heart to pick up more oxygen from the lungs. The pathway of the veins roughly follows that of the arteries, but in reverse, because the blood is coming back to the heart this time. An important detour is taken by some veins into which the capillaries of the small intestine…the major site of food absorption…. merge. The now nutrient-rich veins go through the portal vein to the liver which is the body's "factory". The liver detoxifies poisonous substances, adds important nutrients and other things like proteins and hormones to, and generally does a quality check on, the blood. Then arterioles combine once more to become venules, then finally the hepatic vein. This vein drains into the inferior vena cava, carrying its recently acquired nutritional stores to the right heart, the lungs for an oxygen charge, and back out again through the left heart and great arteries to resume its function of resupplying cells with food and oxygen and carrying off their waste. Meanwhile other veins from other parts of the body are also entering either the vein called the superior vena cava, which drains the upper torso and head. These other veins, however, have not been enriched with nutrients and other substances as have those arising from the upper gut and draining into the inferior vena cava.. WE will go into more detail later on the fascinating arrangements in the gut which allow us to break down a greasy pizza or tortilla into basic nutrients to be gobbled up by our body's cells.

Normal changes in an aging circulatory system

Several decades ago, while doing research on infectious disease in the Guatemalan highlands, our group of researchers was invited to a feast by the hospitable and generous Mayan villagers with whom we worked. The people were poor to a degree we had never seen elsewhere. The chickens they slaughtered for us as their honored guests were so anorexic that little meat was to be found on their tiny limbs and wings. Anecdotally, though, our Mayan hosts had almost no cardiovascular disease, and had no experience with the symptoms of stroke or heart attack, even among their elders. These people had a very hardscrabble but very active lifestyle, trying to get their squash, corn and other crops to grow on a steep mountainside. Many of their children died early of infectious diseases, perhaps another reason cardiovascular disease was rare among them. However, another contributing factor may have been lifestyle. They also had no exposure to processed, calorie rich food, and never, from childhood onward, failed to go up and down their mountainside daily. Of course, their story is anecdotal, and no cardiovascular research had then been done to substantiate our observations.

But we all know that, at least in technologically advanced cultures, cardiovascular disease is perhaps the biggest killer of elderly persons. What is it that happens to the great network of arteries, capillaries, veins, the heart and to a certain extent the lymphatic system that makes it falter in its role as the great nutritional highway we need to deliver oxygen and food to every cell in our body? Assuming that a person has not been born with a congenital heart condition, where the whole system is derailed by misplaced or floppy valves or holes which should have closed before or at birth, the changes of aging happen sooner or later to most of us.

You remember those four chambers of the heart. The right side of the heart, which pumps blood to the lungs, has an easier task than does the left side, where the left atrium receives freshly oxygenated blood from the lungs, passes this blood through the mitral valve to that herculean pumping chamber, the left ventricle, The powerful left ventricle then contracts, sending blood to the most hidden recesses of the body. In the aging process, the right heart changes little, but the left atrium enlarges, and the left ventricle stiffens and thickens. (Up to Date: Normal Aging, George E. Taffet, MD, PP8-10) The aortic and mitral valves in the left heart, whose task it is to preventing any backwash of blood as it is being propelled forward, themselves thicken and can develop calcifications which could cause problems with the electrical conducting system of the heart . Those pacemaker cells in the heart's conduction system drop out at about the rate of 10% a decade! In fact, both muscle cells and cells in the heart's electrical conducting system may apoptose, or drop out of existence. Then too, the maximum rate of contraction that a heart can achieve decreases with age, though the resting heart rate stays pretty much normal.

A significant reason that the left ventricle hypertrophies, or gets thicker and bigger, is that the once compliant blood vessels through which it has to pump blood, themselves actually also stiffen and become less flexible, increasing the work of the left ventricle. These arteries, once young and compliant, develop thickening and rigidity due to actual structural changes! And all this happens even in the absence of atherosclerosis, although disease in the coronary arteries, which supply blood to the heart muscle itself, is found at autopsy in about 75% of men. This disease happens about 2 decades later in women whose premenopausal hormones seem to offer protection.

Keeping the heart pumping well into old age

Choosing your parents wisely: heredity and the circulatory system

Genetics is a rapidly expanding field, and we will be learning a lot more about the genetic underpinnings of cardiovascular disease now that the human genome has been mapped and genetic testing has become much cheaper and more available. However, much other medical information is available and has been for decades. A family history in which one or both parents have had earlier than expected cardiovascular disease increases risk. Concomitantly, increased bad or LDL and VLDL cholesterol increase cardiovascular risk, a fact which has been known for a long time, and now these tests have been genetically refined even further.

Additionally, many genetic and chromosomal diseases are known to increase cardiovascular risk. For example, Turner's syndrome where girls have only one "X" chromosome, and Brugada's disease, first identified in young men in Southeast Asia dying suddenly of arrhythmias, are two of many such conditions. We also know now that being born too big or too small for the time one has spent in the womb can predispose to conditions like hypertension and obesity that in turn set the stage for heart disease. Expect knowledge about the underpinnings of cardiovascular disease to explode in the next few years and decades!

Choosing your environment wisely: Where not to live, what not to eat

Most of us are very aware that sodas and fast foods lead to earlier that acceptable morbidity and mortality. Severe Covid19 infection is now known to be more common in the obese! We are also attuned to the fact that stress can provoke circulatory damage. Poverty can be a big stress, and usually also involves living in unhealthy places such as near freeways or contaminated landfills, or in higher crime areas, or even in homeless camps. Let's not forget lack of exercise, a growing threat for children who prefer electronics to old fashioned outside play. Or smoking, be it cigarettes, marijuana, or possibly Hookahs or vaping. There is even a syndrome called the "broken heart syndrome" also known as stress induced cardiomyopathy. It is thought that this illness may be due to weakened left ventricular pumping with decreased output of oxygen rich blood, or perhaps coronary artery spasm. Either way, it can present with symptoms like those of a heart attack. It is triggered by a sudden, usually emotional shock. Of course, common parlance has referred to dying of a broken heart long before this possibility was reported scientifically.

"Wilbur" was a middle-aged man with a beautiful wife and two children. When his coronary arteries, those blood vessels responsible for bringing blood and oxygen to the mighty heart muscle, got critically blocked. He had to undergo surgery to have them kept open through placement of a stent. He saw quite clearly the two paths opening before him. One path led up a mountain of challenges, the second was much easier and required no change in lifestyle. Wilbur knew the second path would lead to obesity, physical deterioration, a narrowing of his world, and of course inability to keep his wife happy. So Wilbur chose the path up the mountain…quite literally. Over time, he lost his excess fat, stopped all his bad sedentary habits, and started climbing the beautiful mountains that surrounded his home. As he grew older, his heart functionally grew "younger", not because of a reversal of the inevitable changes of aging, but because it was a muscle. Muscles generally respond quite favorably when given the opportunity to function as they were meant to. Let it be said that Wilbur's heart muscle was rehabilitated slowly and thoughtfully. Now Wilbur has another gleam in his eye. In his early sixties, he is actually looking with longing at Mount Everest! His wife? She started exercising too, and now no one would ever guess she is fifty!

Wilbur's story, and that of other strongly motivated people, illustrates the need for lifelong fitness. It also illustrates the fact that some human beings can make impressive changes with the proper motivation. But what about people who don't find themselves so motivated?

There are many "Wilbur's" among seniors, but most older folk, often plagued with aching joints and dilapidated muscles, are not motivated to make the effort to mitigate the cardiovascular changes of aging. Some have cardiovascular issues so severe that adjustments in activity and in the environment, and even the use of medications with real downsides, are inevitable. What are some of these handicapping conditions?

Sig-alerts in the Circulatory System: Damage to the heart muscle: heart attacks, arrhythmias and other roadblocks

The conducting system of the heart, (see above), those electrical impulses from the heart which tell the heart muscle when to contract and beat, like any electrical wiring system, tends towards having cells, especially those in the pivotal sinoatrial and in the atrioventricular nodes, just drop out. Both areas act somewhat as transducers and pick up signals from hormones like epinephrine and some medications like beta blockers which modify heart rate. When the "wiring system" of the heart frays, the upper chamber, or atrium, may go on automatic. The sequential contraction of the atria and ventricles when it no longer functions well, does not give the atria time to fill properly, which of course means the ventricles won't get their usual share of blood, and so the oxygenated blood going to the body will diminish and cells won't get their needed share of energy and oxygen. Like Mr. Lopez, patients will feel fatigued, unable to go about their normal daily activities, unable to walk up a flight of stairs, or even eat properly. Like Mr. L, a 60 year old who presented for a physical exam for what he thought was old age but was really rhythm problem called atrial fibrillation.

But wait! Atrial fibrillation has another mean trick up its sleeve. There is a little side chamber off the left atrium, called the atrial appendage. It probably functions as a kind of "pop-off valve" for increased left ventricular pressure, but the blood in this backwater appendage often clots in persons who have ongoing atrial fibrillation. The clot then can travel through the mitral valve to the left ventricle, out through the aorta and up to the brain, where it can cause a stroke. To combat this tendency for dangerous clots to form, older patients are often put on blood thinning medications. These medications are fairly effective at preventing stroke but increase the risk of bleeding in other areas like the stomach or even from a small cut. One of the clot-busting medications commonly used is called warfarin and requires very close monitoring of the diet because certain healthy foods like some vegetables and salads, change the activity of warfarin, making it either too strong or too weak. In turn, folks on this medication have to be careful to read labels or know what is in the foods they eat when dining out. Some medications also interfere with warfarin. Patients must check out even over the counter medications. There are also newer medications on the market to "thin blood" but all have some precautions attached.

Lastly, some cases of atrial fibrillation can be treated with a procedure called defibrillation, using electricity to shock the heart into a regular rhythm again. There are strict criteria for when where and who is eligible. Some forms of atrial fibrillation are also amenable to surgery.

Heart attacks

Mr. Z was your typical hard charging business man who came to an urgent care clinic with crushing anterior chest pain radiating up to his jaw and down his left arm, nauseous and with considerable anxiety. He was sweating although the day wasn't hot for Southern California. He had driven himself to the facility, because as a take-charge male, he didn't want to upset his wife. The surprise was that with his classical heart attack (or myocardial infarct) symptoms, his electrocardiogram, a crucial test which gives important information about the function of the heart's electrical conduction system and therefore parts of this system that would be changed due to a lack of blood from the infarcted coronary arteries, was totally normal. It is true that other rare problems, like infection or fluid in the sack surrounding the heart, called the pericardial sac, can give similar symptoms. Furthermore, in cases where the electrocardiogram is normal, blood tests are available which can show the loss of function of heart muscle cells whose coronary artery blood supply has very recently been shut off. However, these tests take time, especially at an urgent care facility where blood tests usually have to be sent elsewhere.

But the physician and nurse taking care of Mr. Z had a strong suspicion that he was having a heart attack, and while waiting for confirmatory blood tests, got another electrocardiogram. Sure enough, this one showed the heart attack. Mr. Z was whisked off to the university hospital, had immediate heart surgery, and did very well indeed.

Mrs. L, an African American school teacher, was not so lucky. An intelligent, slim lady only in her mid-fifties, she had a family history of both elevated blood pressure and elevated lipids, the latter being substances in the blood and elsewhere like some forms of cholesterol and like triglycerides. These substances have been associated with the formation of elevated plaques on the insides of blood vessels (endometrial cell lining) which can narrow their diameter and when ruptured, can attract blood clotting substances like platelets that will completely block the artery. If this process of rupture and vessel occlusion happens in one of the coronary arteries feeding the heart muscle, the event becomes a heart attack. Sometimes, if serious narrowing of the coronary blood vessels is seen on arteriography, often done when a person has angina chest pain, that person can have a procedure like a CABG, where a vein from the leg replaces the critically narrowed segment of the involved coronary artery or where an artery called the internal mammary artery is diverted, surgically replacing the blocked segment of that coronary artery. Another procedure to correct the narrowed coronary artery is called percutaneous coronary angioplasty (PCA) where a small balloon is introduced by a guidewire into the affected coronary artery. The balloon then is inflated to compress the obstructing plaque blockage and open up the blood vessel . A stent is then placed in the now opened coronary artery. This stent holds the coronary artery open, hopefully for years!

Mrs. L, with a past history of a heart attack and of a PCA, was closely followed by her cardiologist. However, one day she took a train trip to visit her son. In spite of everything which had been done to prevent it, this kindly lady died of a fatal heart attack on her trip back home. Her death still saddens her family and health care providers.

What to do immediately

Advanced cardiac life support classes teach that calling for help through 911 for paramedic support is the most important intervention for symptoms of cardiovascular disease such as a heart attack or a stroke. Recognition, especially of the warning signs of a cerebrovascular attack (CVA), requires a bit of knowledge. Symptoms of a CVA can include numbness, weakness, tingling or paralysis of face or extremities, often involving one half of the body only, and/or loss of speech, even seizures or unconsciousness. Heart attack symptoms can involve severe mid-chest pressure like "an elephant sitting on my chest", nausea, pain radiating to neck or usually the left arm, sweating weakness and in women especially, more nonclassical symptoms, sometimes gastrointestinal. Taking a basic cardiovascular life support class is always a good option. If you are going to have a heart attack, Seattle is the place to have it. Due to intensive public education, this city has the highest survival rate of any city in the country.

Making a damaged heart better: medication, surgery and other interventions, lifestyle

African American women are at increased risk of cardiovascular disease, and cardiovascular disease claims more women's as well as men's lives than other diagnoses. Cardiovascular mortality is highest in African Americans and interestingly is also high in some sub-Saharan countries, including Sudan (237.35 deaths per 100,000), Ghana (155.08 deaths per 100,000) and Nigeria (117.12 deaths per 100,000) . (14) (WHO death rate per 100,000 from CVD, Age-adjusted death rates, 2017). The next highest rate is in non-Hispanic US whites, followed by Hispanic Americans, Native Americans and lastly Asian/Pacific Islanders, a very heterogeneous grouping. In fact, in Americans older than 65, women suffer more cardiovascular events numerically than do men!

Cardiologists worldwide have introduced amazing technologic and drug interventions into our armamentarium, though they have not reversed the changes of aging. Many seniors live with cardiovascular diseases of various sorts, chronic coronary artery disease being one of the most common.

Most of these patients, like Mr. G, present with fatigue or shortness of breath, though some get characteristic chest pain primarily when engaged in strenuous activity. Mr. G. had both. An avid runner at 71, this Asian- American male prided himself on his early morning jogs. He constantly pushed himself to run faster and faster. That is when he started having typical chest pressure after he'd run a couple of miles. He put off seeking care or decreasing his pace for a couple of months. The pressure persisted, and eventually he arrived at the door of his cardiologist. Patients like Mr. G are often put through a battery of testing, the firs being an exercise stress test. Mr. G was in good physical shape generally, so his treadmill stress test was positive at a fairly impressive level of exercise. A treadmill stress test is done with a patient exercising while continuously being monitored by electrocardiogram for signs of compromised coronary blood flow. Blood pressure is also checked during the procedure, and treadmill speed can be increased to challenge the heart's ability to cope. Pharmacologic stress tests can be done for persons unable to run on a treadmill.

In these pharmacologic tests, medications to increase stress on the heart are given to check for insufficient coronary blood flow. Echocardiograms are rather like the ultrasounds we do to check on babies in utero. In the case of echocardiograms, the cardiologist can see how the heart muscle contracts, how thick the chambers are, how the heart valves are working, or even if some of the heart muscle is being deprived of blood due to a blocked coronary blood vessel. Lastly, percutaneous angiography provides very precise information about the status of coronary blood vessels. In this process, which can be coupled with correction of the blocked coronary artery when it is identified better, a catheter is placed in the groin artery (femoral) threaded up to the heart and maneuvered to where the coronary arteries come off the aortic sinus (beginning of aorta as it exits from the left ventricle of the heart). If a block is identified in a coronary artery, coronary angioplasty can be done then and there. Centers that have 24/7 availability to do percutaneous coronary angiography are doing so for acute heart attack patients, thereby speeding recovery and saving lives. Another improvement, if immediate access to the coronary arteries is not needed, is the CT coronary angiogram, which doesn't involve catheter introduction.

Back to Mr. G. In his case, medical treatment with drugs protecting the heart, initially sufficed, and he modified his running protocol, doing well. Medical treatment of angina can also be used for very elderly or sick persons who would not be able to tolerate the stress of some of the above interventions.

Heart failure itself, (CHF) often due in the elderly to coronary artery disease, is the most common cause of elder hospitalization and of disability. When Mr. A came back from an annual national conference for Sociology Professors, he was clearly in distress. A large diabetic man, he had chronic congestive heart failure and morbid obesity, was mobile only through use of his specially constructed scooter, but at age 63, was a favorite college professor. His congestive heart failure, which had presented with shortness of breath, excessive tiredness, and swelling of his already massive legs, was well controlled at home with diet and medication. His very attentive wife and excellent cardiologist made sure his diet was controlled, although a bit unappetizing, and his medications were taken on time and effective. Unfortunately, his professional conference presented him with an unsupervised opportunity to eat salted foods, down soft drinks, and generally run amuk food wise. He also forgot to take his medications half the time. When he got home from the four day meeting, he was several pounds heavier, decidedly short of breath, edematous, and was immediately carted off by Mrs. A to see his doctor. He plans not to attend any more national conferences, (at least not without his wife).

Most deaths due to heart failure occur in persons above 75. However, heart failure is a major cause of disability, loss of independence and the ability to care for one's own needs, and of admittance to long term care facilities. (Geriatric Review syllabus, 9th edition) Besides the aging of heart and blood vessels, and of course heredity, other more reversible causes are hypertension, obesity, lifelong habits like smoking, dietary malfeasance and drugs. In fact, things that happen to a fetus in utero, it is suggested, may predispose to the conditions that make congestive heart failure more likely much later in life.

There are a collection of physical complaints that may make a health care professional look for congestive heart failure. In addition to leg edema, these may include needing to sleep on a pile of pillows to breathe well at night, or even having to get up at night and go to a window to catch one's breath! On exam, neck veins may be engorged (swollen with backed up blood) and the liver larger than normal. The physical exam, EKG showing enlargement and thickness of the left ventricle, blood tests and finally such tests as the echocardiogram may solidify a diagnosis suspected on exam. In the absence of a surgical or other interventional remedy or of the use of an implantable pacemaker, lifestyle changes and medications become the backbone of treatment. Because of the limitations in activity, environmental interventions may also be in order.

When the heart's wiring is getting "frayed" as a person ages, causing unexpected and dangerous irregularities in heart rhythm and subsequently the heart's pumping ability, other interventions are in order. If the heart is not pumping normally, people can feel very fatigued, faint and fall causing injury, or even die. A variety of implantable electronic devices called pacemakers are available to treat the specific rhythm disturbance, or arrhythmia identified through a sophisticated array of testing. Some cardiologists even specialize in this specific area of heart disease. Pacemakers come in a variety of flavors and makes. Pacemakers use electrical pulses to help the heart pump at a normal rate. (NIH-National heart, lung and blood institute) Most pacemakers are used if someone's heart rate is too slow (bradycardia), or is erratic. Some defibrillators will give a big electric shock if the heart stops.

Changes in the Arteries with Aging and Bad Habits: Downstream effects of poor arterial circulation

A word about the blood vessels, which also undergo changes as we age. They generally become thickened and more tortuous or twisty. They also develop plaques of atherosclerosis, known as hardening of the arteries, similar to the changes that can occur in the coronary arteries which lead to heart attacks. Aneurisms can develop in the aorta and other arteries. Aneurisms are weak areas in the wall of the blood vessel leading to ballooning of the side of the vessel. Then the blood vessel can dissect, sending blood along the layers of the wall of the blood vessel, or even rupture, which usually leads to rapid death unless immediately addressed surgically with lightning speed.

Perhaps the greatest risk for getting an aneurism, especially of the aorta, is being a smoker. But if blood vessels are blocked severely in the legs, for example, this can lead to tissue death and the need for amputation. Fortunately, if detected early enough, revascularization of the blood vessels in the pelvis, where the aorta divides in two, creating the common iliac arteries which supply the legs and other structures, is sometimes possible.

What do all these changes in circulation mean for seniors? The aging of the heart and of the circulatory system mean that there is less reserve when disease occurs. For example, pneumonia in an older person frequently triggers arrhythmias or even heart failure. When circulatory failure reaches a critical point, the ability to maintain function in other organs, like the kidneys, is lost. This results in a domino effect on the entire body. The impact is felt far and wide, on family function, on social services, and even on architectural design. One seventy-year-old, building a home for his new bride of sixty-five, installed elevators to make his life easier and hers also as she presumably would be the one caring for him as he grew older.

When to suspect poor circulation: suspicious behavior and complaints

Mr. B, a 74-year-old male, came in to see the physician with a chip on his shoulder. Viagra hadn't worked, he couldn't get a good erection. What would his physician do about this situation, he challenged. Surely medical science had an answer, and he needed it quickly. Unfortunately, ED may have a circulatory origin. After exploring other etiologies, hardening of the penile artery and more widespread atherosclerosis needs to be investigated. Likewise, numbness in the feet, or a transient episode of stroke-like neurologic symptoms should make a person take a good look at his or her circulation. Health care providers often check for the pulses in the feet because often, and especially in diabetes, these are the pulses that show signs of wear and tear or even very poor blood flow. Similarly, pressure on skin tells one if there may be vascular disease. A slow return of the normal pink color may be a warning sign of poor perfusion. The arteries in the legs are often affected by poor circulation and atherosclerosis. Classic symptoms include getting leg pain after walking a block or two, and having this pain go away after resting, only to return when an identical distance is traversed. This symptom of peripheral arterial disease is called intermittent claudication. If blood flow to the legs and feet diminishes even further, critical limb ischemia, causing pain in the foot, nonhealing wounds or even gangrene, can occur. At this juncture, catheter-based balloon angioplasty and stenting, akin to what is done for blocked coronary arteries, can be a life and limb saver. Some medications are sometimes used for milder disease in the lower extremity arteries either initially before endo (within) vascular intervention, or as treatment in appropriate cases.

Most of all, stop smoking!

What can be done to improve the health of peripheral arteries

Reduction in cholesterol, cessation of smoking, a good diet can go a long way towards stopping progression of the arteries and arterioles. Revascularization, such as is done for the coronary arteries, can also be done on key peripheral arteries. Exercise done early in the course of blockage on a regular and progressive basis, allows the legs to grow blood vessels which will bypass the obstructed ones, kind of like taking a road detour, and once again bring nourishing blood to tissues. See also the above discussion about stenting .

Problems with the veins

Venous disease isn't quite as critical as arterial disease. However, it too can cause complicated problems. Lets take a look at how the veins, tasked with return of poorly oxygenated blood back to the heart, are constructed. As you recall this blood has just given up its oxygen to individual cells as it traversed to capillary beds.

The veins are thinner and less elastic than are the arteries. They have internal valves that keep the blood returning to the heart from backwashing, Although all veins are tasked with returning blood to the heart, and most veins connect with the right side of the heart, the pulmonary veins are an exception, because they carry blood freshly oxygenated in the lungs back to the left side of the heart, to be distributed by the powerful left ventricle to the arteries.

Then there is the portal vein. This vein carries nutrient- rich blood from the small intestine's absorptive structures to the liver. The liver is the body's "factory", Among other duties, it is tasked with processing the nutrients, or food, absorbed from the small intestine and removing any toxic substances that may have accompanied these nutrients, Following its trip through the liver, the venous blood, now rich in processed food molecules, gets back to the right atrium, thence to the right ventricle and through the pulmonary artery to the lungs.

Thus this two circuit system of arteries and veins, connected by tiny capillary beds, continuously supplies food and oxygen to all the cells in the body.

Varicose veins: causes. Complaints and treatment

Two major issues that have to do with the veins are increasingly common as people grow older. The first, and most common, is the occurrence of varices, especially in the legs and feet but also elsewhere in the body. Varices are swollen veins whose valves have failed, usually in the legs and feet, although they can even involve other areas, even the genitals.

Maybelle had had quite a few pregnancies in the day, had grown large after menopause, and didn't like to exercise. Over time. She developed ugly varicose veins, but comforted herself with the fact that her mother and grandmother had coped with these ugly bluish vessels popping out on their lower legs too. Then she began to notice darker discoloration in the area above her ankles. She refused to wear the tight thigh high stockings her doctor suggested, and just couldn't remember to elevate her legs above heart level several times a day as instructed. However, when she developed a nonhealing venous stasis ulcer above her lateral right ankle, she became more alarmed. Finally, she agreed to a consult with wound management specialists, but it took months and expert help, Unna boot placement and eventually sclerotherapy to curb her unruly veins. As mentioned above, veins have valves to keep returning blood flowing towards the heart. The muscles of the legs also help squeeze the returning venous blood upward. Several factors can disrupt the function of the valves in the veins, especially in the legs. Varicose veins in the legs tend to be genetic in some families. Though both males and females can develop varicosities especially in the legs, uterine pressure during repeated pregnancies may also be a factor in causing venous dilatation, or widening in diameter, and in disrupting the delicate venous valvular structures. Back pressure can cause unsightly swelling of the legs Packing on pounds, and not exercising seems to play a role also in the creation of varicose veins. With the development of significant leg varicosities, people often complain of leg heaviness, aching when standing, and swelling or edema, especially at the end of the day. Once an ulcer develops, however, healing may take months, and debriding dead tissue and fibrin will often be needed on a regular basis to permit good new granulation tissue to help close the ulcer. Sometimes even grafting is necessary.

Deep vein thrombosis: clots leading to the heart, lungs and other important places

Unsightly and disabling though varicose veins may be, a more lethal problem is the development of a blood clot inside the vein (or rarely in an artery). There is a delicate balance that keeps our blood flowing freely in our vascular system, but that causes our blood to clot when a cut happens. A complicated cascade of chemical reactions is set in motion when a vein or artery, or arteriole is cut or opened. This process protects us from bleeding to death from injuries. However, should this cascade be activated within a blood vessel, spontaneously, occlusion of the blood vessel will cause trouble downstream. In the case of a deep vein thrombosis, which usually occurs in the leg but can occur elsewhere, the clot can break off, travel upward to the lungs and cause a pulmonary embolus or lung clot. If this clot in the veins going to the lung is massive enough, blood will not get to the lung tissue to be oxygenated, and death will ensue.

Risk factors for getting clots in the veins

As we grow older, the balance between free flow of blood in the blood vessels and clotting when needed seems sometimes to swing a bit in the direction of clotting.

Mr. B was a guy who at age 60 was retired from a series of menial jobs and didn't really do much except watch TV. He was friendly and got along well with everyone, but had never had intellectual aspirations, and barely squeaked by in school. He rented a room from elderly but spry woman, who would frequently include him in her dinner plans. Life was good. Then one day, after being particularly sedentary for quite a while, he developed swelling, warmth and tenderness in his left leg. Walking was especially painful. However, when he developed shortness of breath, it was time to go to the local emergency department, where a blood test (D-dimer) was suggestive, an ultrasound study of the leg was equivocal, and a lung scan (ventilation/perfusion) was indeterminate. He was transported to another hospital where pulmonary angiography (contrast study of the pulmonary arteries) gave a definitive diagnosis of a pulmonary embolus. He was later found to have a genetic mutation which made his blood clot more easily that it should. He was immediately put on a blood thinner, or anticoagulant, encouraged to change his lifestyle to a more active one, and has done well for years. Being the "nice guy" that he is, he is very adherent to his medication and hardly ever misses his medical visits. Interestingly, a review of family history disclosed another family member who had a history of a deep vein thrombosis, and probably had a similar genetic mutation.

Besides different types of genetic mutations causing an increased tendency towards blood clotting, and the aging process itself, some other factors that increase clotting risk in older adults include hospitalization and nursing home residence, central venous catheters, surgery, trauma, chronic lung disease, having relatives who had clots and even certain medications, especially hormone replacement therapy. Having a prior occurrence oneself will be a worry for future events. (15) Geriatri Review Syllabus, 9th edition) Many cancers substantially raise the risk of clot formation. One other real risk is stasis, or not moving around. This is why long automobile trips, and especially long airplane trips, are especially risky.

Medical approach

Suspicion of a deep vein thrombosis is usually aroused by clinical complaints. Mr. B had o swelling, warmth, pain and tenderness in the leg, without other obvious cause such as a cellulitis infection. A family or personal history, the presence of one or more predisposing factors, and of lack of activity will elevate suspicion. A blood test called a d-dimer, when abnormal, l can raise probability but indicates the need for further testing. An ultrasound (sound wave test) may reveal a clot. Additional symptoms like shortness of breath and occasionally EKG changes or changes in oxygenation of blood will mandate further evaluation for a clot which has traveled to the lung (pulmonary embolus) Tests like a ventilation-perfusion lung scan or spiral CT of the chest are useful if definitive. Pulmonary arteriography is the gold standard. Prevention of future clots demands lifestyle changes, and the use of one of a selection of "clot busters", or anticoagulants, sometimes for life! Anticoagulants have their own risks and the selection of one over another, as well as length of use, becomes an important clinical decision.

High Blood Pressure: the cardiovascular system's major foe

High blood pressure is a term that gets a lot of press, and with good reason. It describes an excess of force pushing against the walls of arteries. An analogy would be a garden hose subjected to super high-water pressure. Over time, the garden hose might weaken, or even leak However, our arteries are living tissue, and unlike a garden hose, can expand or contract in diameter when needed. Unfortunately, as we grow older, this versatility diminishes. Our arteries become more rigid. Systolic blood pressure (measuring the heart's "push"or the force of active contraction) can become higher, while the diastolic (run-off blood pressure) sometimes diminishes.

What controllable factors increase blood pressure?

Other processes like the buildup of plaque cholesterol can further damage the innards of blood vessels over time.. Blood pressure changes from minute to minute: it is not a static measurement. Hormones, drugs like caffeine and even cold remedies like Sudafed (pseudoephedrine) among many others, can increase blood pressure. Exercise can transiently increase blood pressure, although the overall effect of regular exercise is to lower resting blood pressure. Chronic use of substances like alcohol, of many illegal drugs like cocaine and amphetamines, and even muscle building substances like creatine also have a bad effect on blood pressure. Besides medications, many other factors can increase blood pressure, including chronic stress, inappropriate diets especially those containing foods with excess salt, certain types of congenital heart disease, hormonal influences, and unfortunately, one's heredity. Persons of African ancestry often have variations in certain hormones which make them especially susceptible to the diseases that can result from chronic hypertension. Surveillance is especially important and actually should start in childhood.

Most health care providers have patients who have had hypertension resulting in heart attacks or strokes in their 20's or 30's from the effects of drugs like cocaine and amphetamines. This is such a potent risk factor that one inner city hospital used to do drug screens on just about every patient presenting with cardiovascular symptoms, and found many folks. Some quite elderly, had illegal drugs in their systems! The oldest was actually 91!

Why is hypertension called the "silent killer"?

When high blood pressure, or hypertension, has existed over many decades, damage is ongoing, and often has no symptoms till something catastrophic, like a stroke or heart attack occurs. This is why hypertension is called the "silent killer." Autopsies done on young soldiers during the Korean War actually showed the buildup of cholesterol streaks in arteries in these wartime casualties who were barely out of high school. These streaks become elevations called plaque or atheroma, and their occurrence, along with high blood pressure, are thought to be the processes responsible for most heart attacks.

Diagnosis of Hypertension

Sally always thought that hypertension was the end result of dealing with stress. It seemed perfectly plausible. You were angry, frustrated, anxious, and your blood pressure went up. That is why she was not surprised when her doctor told her that she was developing hypertension. Her daughter had a drug problem, and Sally was given custody her four grandchildren ranging in age from 5 months through 4 years. Talk about stress! Sally presumed that when her daughter got through rehab, and once again resumed her duties as a mother, her hypertension would melt away. Not so, her physician explained. The diagnosis of hypertension is based on physiology, and is made by taking successive measurements of blood pressure under controlled conditions over time. Hypertension is also age specific. Blood pressures which would be normal in an adult are considered abnormal in a child and are referenced to the child's age, height and sex.(16) (The Harriet Lane Handbook, A manual for pediatric house officers. The Johns Hopkins Hospital, Editors M. Tschudy and K.Arcara, Elsevier, Multiple Editions) Blood pressure considered in the hypertensive range also vary by age and disease in adults. For example, blood pressure in a person with diabetes should generally be kept lower than in a non-diabetic since hypertension aggravates the cardiovascular effects of diabetes. Some people have so-called "white coat hypertension" and need blood pressures taken at home to get accurate readings…please see below. There are two readings taken when measuring blood pressure. The systolic blood pressure measures the heart's peak pumping push, and the diastolic pressure measures "run-off" pressure when the ventricles are not contracting actively. The pulse pressure is the lower diastolic blood pressure subtracted from the higher systolic pressure.

Sometimes a person will come in with such a high blood pressure that lowering the pressure becomes an emergency. Taking several readings over time is impractical. A heart attack or stroke could occur in between measurements. If symptoms of an impending catastrophe are found, that person would be treated expediciously in an emergency setting with intravenous mediations. Luckily, this is a rare event.

Medications for controlling hypertension: the good, the bad and the ugly

There are several medications which can be very helpful in lowering blood pressure, and some also help with other intertwined diseases. For example, classes of drugs called ACE's and ARBs are helpful in preserving kidney health and filtering ability at the same time as they reduce blood pressure. Since all drugs have rare side effects, these must be watched for, and if they occur, persons can be switched to other blood pressure medications better individualized for them. Ms., C, a sixty something year old quite obese lady, was on one of the "ACE" drugs for a year or more both because of her elevated blood pressure and because her blood sugar was creeping up. She did very well until one day, for unknown reasons, her lips and tongue started swelling, The swelling advanced pretty rapidly, she went to the ER. There, a specialist in otolaryngology couldn't figure out what had triggered her problem, known as angioedema. Finally, it was determined that her ACE medication may have been the cause. A handful of other cases had been reported, but usually when the drug was first started. Nonetheless, Ms.C was taken off her ACE, and her symptoms resolved completely. Ms. C's experience was a very rare side effect of this class of medication, but vigilance is always appropriate with any medication. Especially in seniors, who have less reserve, and who are often on several drugs, any unusual changes always require checking medications first.

However, treatment of high blood pressure has saved many lives by preventing the sequalae of stroke, heart attack, and even such rare problems as ischemic bowel disease. In this disease, hardening of the arteries processing food which increases the demand for blood in the digestive system, causes severe pain. Think of this process as being analogous to a heart attack in the belly!

When is hypertension not hypertension?

Since blood pressure can vary from moment to moment, and since going to see one's doctor is stress producing, there is a common entity called "white coat hypertension". Blood pressure measured in a medical setting is quite high, but in a person's daily life, the blood pressure is perfectly normal. When this problem is suspected, people are often sent home with their own blood pressure equipment and told to take their blood pressure reading at various times during their waking day. If these readings are normal, only lifestyle improvement, like not eating fast foods, avoiding excessive salting of foods, looking into stresses that could be reduced a bit, and exercising daily, are in order, as they are for all of us. (occasionally, a new health care provider is in order)

Helping seniors take their medications as ordered.

It was so frustrating for Mr. E's nurse practitioner. No matter how many blood pressure medications she added or changed in a desperate attempt to regulate his blood pressure, nothing worked. She tried giving him a home blood pressure cuff. He invariably "forgot" to bring in his readings. His nurse practitioner suspected that he hadn't checked his blood pressure at home and was too embarrassed to tell her. Finally, in desperation, after laying out all the bad things that could happen if Mr. E didn't comply with the plan of treatment, the nurse practitioner asked if Mrs. could be present at the next visit. Mrs. E, the problem solver of the family, promptly bought a 7 day medicine container and made sure it was filled every Sunday after church, and put in a place the grandchildren couldn't reach when they visited. She also made sure the clock on her husband's smart phone was set to 9 am, by which time he would have put in his hearing aids. If he hadn't taken his meds and checked and recorded his blood pressure, well, the consequences would be dire, and he knew it. Problem solved!

Heart Failure

What heart failure is and how to recognize it: different types and presentations

Heart failure can best be described as inability of the pumping mechanism of the heart to meet the demands of the body's cells for oxygen and nourishment. The New York Heart Association has a classification of severity by symptoms as follows:

Class I: no limitation of normal activities

Class II: mild shortness of breath, slight limitation during normal activity

Class III: marked limitation of activities eg: walking short distances

Class IV: symptoms even at rest (Specifications Manual for Joint Commission National Quality Measure (V2016A)

Mr . Z was a longtime patient. He was a fairly active guy, did yard work, walked a lot and collected used ammo from the local shooting range for recycling. He had a known history of a leaky aortic valve, but his cardiologist kept an eye on him every 6 months or so. One day he came in complaining of "having to slow down a bit" . This complaint didn't fit his youngish age, or his personality. On examination, he had swelling of his lower legs, his liver was a bit larger than on previous visits, and his heart murmur was getting decidedly noisier. His cardiologist was called, saw him that very week, and sent him to a cardiovascular surgeon. But Mr. Z was scared of the surgery to fix his very leaky aortic heart valve, which was backflowing and making it impossible for his heart to put out enough blood for his actively metabolizing muscles when he walked or did "weed whacking". However, he reluctantly agreed to have the surgery, which would be done via his artery, when he heard the tale of Mr. Q.

Mr. Q was a farmer and had a large number of children. He also had a history of aortic insufficiency, same as Mr. Z. His was caused by rheumatic fever as a child and had worsened with age. His symptoms were the same as Mr. Z's. He absolutely refused surgery, because there was no one else to do the farm work, and all those children had to be fed and clothed. Argument was futile. Mr. Q died suddenly a few months after spring planting.

Most heart failure in our country is not caused by disease of the heart valves, but rather by coronary heart disease. Other causes are viruses or other infections of the heart muscle, (Covid 19 can do this) certain types of infectious processes or fluid collections in the pericardium, which is the sac around the heart muscle, malfunction of the heart valves either from disease or maldevelopment of the heart in utero, tumors, and rarely toxins or other substances which attack the heart muscle.

What a person with heart failure may complain about

People with heart failure just aren't getting enough oxygen to their organs and muscles. Shortness of breath with exercise is a common initial symptom. Leg edema is so common. Since when we lie down for sleep, gravity redistributes the body's fluid, and since our bodies are about 70% water, the lungs may become relatively flooded Persons with heart failure will usually sleep on a bunch of pillows and may awaken from sleep and go to a window to " get more air into" their lungs. Babies who are born with heart anomalies may be very hungry, but after a small amount of milk may get sweaty and refuse further nourishment This is because feeding activity is too strenuous for their weakened hearts. Similarly, older folk may cut back on oral intake, and just not feel like eating. When heart failure becomes severe, a person may get short of breath just sitting.

How heart failure is treated

Causes that can be treated surgically

Many causes of heart failure can be treated surgically, both in infants and children, and in older adults. Newer equipment and devices have enabled cardiothoracic surgeons and interventional cardiologists to repair valves and clogged arteries via vascular access without "cracking the chest" or doing a thoracotomy through the chest. If worse comes to worst, heart transplants are available at some large medical centers, made safer by drugs which prevent the immune system from rejecting the "foreign" heart. Of course there are many complicated issues surrounding all of these interventions, not the least of which is finding enough hearts to transplant and deciding the persons who will be recipients.

Causes usually treated medically

Most heart failure is treated medically with a variety of medications that get rid of excess body fluid, prevent or retard plaque buildup in arteries, relieve pressure on the heart muscle, control high blood pressure, protect the heart from, or treat, preexisting infection as would be the case if a heart valve failed because it got infected with bacteria. Patients must do their part, by religiously taking medications, following dietary directions, getting appropriate exercise when indicated, and of course stopping drugs, alcohol, and tobacco when these contribute to heart failure, The future looks bright for new types of medications being developed, but heart failure is still a very grave cause of mortality especially in older folk.

CHAPTER 6

What Happens to Food: Lips to Exit

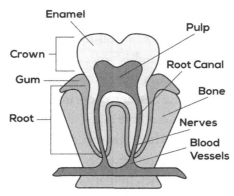

Tooth Anatomy

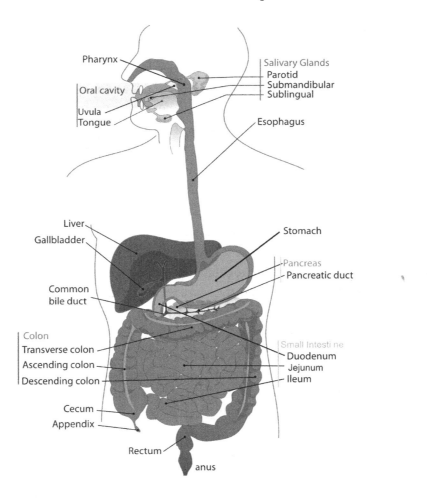

Poor Mr. Z. The few incisors remaining in the front of his mouth hung like swords from his upper jaw, and his diet would have made a one-year-old wince in disgust. His teeth to tattoo ratio, an important "tongue in cheek" marker in the mountains where he'd lived, was about 1 to 20. Yes, Mr. Z had interesting tattoos. However, his gums were receding. His lower jaw, once strong and manly, was gently wasting away. The rest of his body was also feeling the effects of his failing nutrition. He was constipated, his muscles had seen better days, and even his thought processes were becoming sluggish. Mr Z's health problems all began in his teeth, or lack thereof!

The saying goes, that when a man stops talking (or thinking) about his sexual prowess and starts mulling over his ability to defecate successfully, he is getting old. However, successful digestion supports all the other components of healthy living too, especially as one ages, so it is important to know a little bit about how food is processed.

One can think of the digestive tract as a long tube where things happen that enable a thick steak or a helping of cabbage to be converted into odoriferous waste (with some loss of content along the way). In this tube, several processes take place. Various additives mix with food to render it easy to be assimilated into the body. After this processing, the broken-down components of that steak are absorbed through the lining of the tube. Then the cells in the tube's lining have to push the steak's essential molecules into the circulation to be sent to all the hungry cells in the body. More on this process later!

Lifetime of Good Teeth or the oral cavity: not just for kissing!

The oral cavity consists of very important structures whose job it is to start the breakdown process for that steak you love. The lips confine the steak and make chewing socially acceptable. The teeth fit into the upper and lower jawbones and cut the steak into tinier fragments. The alveolar bone of the maxilla and the mandible holds the teeth firmly in place and provides a passageway for the nerves and blood vessels that grow and nourish the teeth. The temporomandibular joint allows the lower jaw to grind against the upper jaw, so the embedded teeth can do their job. Muscles of chewing propel the jaw, while the orofacial muscles permit the lips to act as sealants as well as to activate facial expression. Then there is the mucosa, those cells which line the gums, palate, and cheeks and are studded with mucous glands. The tongue moves food around in the mouth, and lets the eater enjoy the process of eating the steak. In this gustatory capacity, the taste buds are powerfully assisted by the olfactory nerves in the nose. Taste without smell would greatly diminish the pleasure of eating that expensive steak. Then we have the salivary glands, which secrete saliva into the mouth. The parotids wind around the lower ears, and their ducts enter the mouth at the level of the upper second molars. The submental and submaxillary glands nestle below the arches of the mandible. You have probably felt saliva squirting up from under your tongue when you were very hungry and bit into an especially welcome morsel of food. (17) (Chapter 8: Oral health in Elderly People, Michele J. Saunders DDS, MS, MPH and Chih-Ko Yeh, DDS, PP 163-207, JB's pub, Louisville, Ky))

Saliva lubricates food, and also contains substances like antibacterial proteins which control the growth of oral bacteria and neutralize their acid production, all of which protect the teeth over time. But saliva also contains salivary amylase, a very important digestive enzyme that begins the process of breaking down dietary starch and disaccharides in that cabbage, and perhaps the roll that went with the steak so that the nutrients therein can be absorbed.

Mrs. XY had an autoimmune condition known as Sjogrun's syndrome. Her immune cells were attacking the glands that produced saliva and tears. She had tried everything from artificial saliva to swallowing her food by taking a gulp of water with each swallow. Not only was eating a real chore instead of a pleasure, but her teeth, without protective saliva, were rotting away. Her disease was a classical manifestation of immunity run amok!

More about the teeth, whose structure and function is much more complex that might be thought. The teeth snuggle deep in alveolar bone, their roots bound to the alveolar bone by the periodontal ligament. Their hard enamel layer is superimposed on the softer dentine layer and is the part of the tooth we see protruding from the gingiva in healthy young adults. The pulp chamber, lining the interior of the tooth, carries nerves and blood vessels.

A five-year-old girl, upon being taken to a museum housing a collection of lifelike prehistoric and contemporary animals, busied herself with inspecting the dentition of these fierce taxidermist's creatures. She soon figured out that front teeth were for cutting food. The wicked canines she saw on a saber tooth tiger were for ripping through tough carcasses. The grinding molars were useful for an herbivore's diet. A career as a dentist may be in this child's future. Humans, who are both carnivores and herbivores, of course have all these types of teeth.

What happens to teeth and gums as we age

When a baby is learning how to talk, his muscles controlling speech develop from the back of the mouth to the front. This is the reason a two-month-old uses vowels to coo. Sounds like "Ahhh" and "Ohhh" come mostly from the back of the mouth. In almost every culture, babies say "dada" before they say "mama". Yet Mom has done the majority of childcare. Is this linguistic turnabout showing ingratitude on the part of her nine-month-old? Articulating "dada" uses the tongue and the roof of the mouth, whereas "mama" demands the use of the lips. Mastery of the lip muscles occurs after mastery of the more proximal tongue. Certainly, the oral cavity is not only important for nutrition, but also for social communication, Therefore the changes of aging impact not only nutrition, and through nutrition, every other bodily function, but also the maintenance of healthy social interaction.

As we age, several things can happen to our mouth structures that both involve and affect our dentition. The jaw bones resorb and become less resistant to trauma and disease. The gums regress, leaving the substance covering the root surfaces of the teeth, exposed. This surface, or cementum, is less resistant to the acids in soft drinks, to sugars, and to tobacco. Root decay, or caries, develops. Periodontal disease and loss of teeth can then occur. Additionally, as alveolar jaw tissue is lost, implants and dentures become problematic. The blood vessels and nerves in the teeth themselves decline in function, the average human tooth pulp lasting only about the biblical threescore and ten years. Tooth wear is a problem since the enamel, that top shiny hard surface of one's pearly whites, cannot replace itself. With the pulp holding the blood supply and nerves of the tooth also getting older, seniors may become less aware of tooth pain and thus the need for urgent dental care. Then too, pearly whites often have difficulty maintaining their whiteness due to worn enamel and discoloration from bad habits like smoking. Affected teeth will have an unattractive yellow or dark color. Gingival recession exposes more of the tooth surface and root. The periodontal ligaments anchoring the tooth to alveolar bone lose their grip, further loosening the tooth. 9180 (Wanda.C. Gonzalves, MD, A. Stevens Wrightson, MD and Robert G. Henry, DMD, MPH, Common Oral Conditions in Older Persons, American Family Physician, Oct.1, 2008, 78 (7) : 845-852.)

An elderly lady knew how to make friends. She seemed to sense instinctively that the muscles in her face were aging and sagging, and that her facial and chewing musculature in repose gave her an unhappy look. So, she made every effort to smile around people, though smiling took thought and planning at times. Happily, she lived to be 101, and the social interactions her smiling face evoked probably contributed to her longevity.

Why teeth are critical to elder nutrition: diet and avoidance of tooth unfriendly food and drink

Nutrition involves the breakdown and assimilation of proteins, carbohydrates and fats, and the absorption of a smattering of vitamins and minerals. Complex carbohydrates, such as those found in vegetables and fruit, generally require a bit more work to chew, although cooking renders mastication easier. Proteins are the building blocks of tissue, and meat proteins even when cooked, still generally require quite a bit of tooth work. When one's teeth and jaws are no longer functional, nutrition is probably going to suffer.

The Center for Disease Control and Prevention, in its overview entitled "the Oral Health of Older Americans", notes that "there is noticeable social inequality in the oral health of older adults", private dental insurance being usually an out of pocket expense difficult for many on a fixed income to work into their budgets. Also, dental care in an older person is usually more complex. In fact, the CDC reports that older folks below the poverty line report 300% more unmet dental needs than those at or above the poverty line.

Poor teeth complicate the process of ingesting nutrient rich food which can be chewed, leading to poor global health. Older folk with insufficient financial resources to pay for appropriate chewable foods, and with poor dentition, enter a vicious cycle which further perpetuates tooth loss. Perhaps the real solution lies in good oral care from the time those first baby teeth poke their way through the mucosa of the mandible!

CARE OF THE TEETH, THE DENTIST AS FRIEND

Dentists have been the butt of jokes almost as frequently as lawyers. Dental care a generation or two ago was a painful matter. Improvements in dental care and pain prevention have changed that almost as much as the introduction of more efficient drills. People of a certain age may vividly remember the old days and be bit less eager than today's generation in seeking dental care. Many people have not, over a lifetime, brushed and flossed their teeth several times a day, stayed away from evil foods like cola sodas and candies, not to mention cigarettes, and may simply not have the availability of a gerodentist in their communities.

The Anatomy of a Successful Swallow

The part played by structures from the lips to the gastroesophageal sphincter (and yes, the sense of smell)

Imbibing or ingesting is a complicated process which begins in utero. The breastfed newborn works hard for his dinner. He must pull the nipple aureola (the dark red tip of the breast) into the mouth and squeeze the milk out by compressing the nipple against the roof of his mouth. Very young babies have a tongue thrust: food placed on the front part of their tongues will be pushed out. Eventually teeth protrude, mastery is gained over primitive reflexes and a smooth swallow ensues. Here is what happens. During swallowing, the food being corralled in the mouth by the lips is mixed with saliva to begin the digestive process. The anterior tongue and palate work together as swallowing begins to ensure that the bolus of food or fluids is propelled backwards into the back of the mouth or pharynx. Meanwhile the soft palate rises preventing food from going into the nose. Once the food or liquid is in the pharynx, it could theoretically go down or be aspirated into the trachea or windpipe. However a structure appended to the glottis, called the epiglottis, assisted by the rising larynx or voice box, shuts off the trachea, allowing the food or liquid to travel safely down the esophagus to get to the stomach. This complex activity demands the coordination of half of the cranial nerves, a large number of the muscles of the head and neck, their activity sequenced appropriately, and of course cerebral input into the medullary swallow center, the instigation of swallowing being of course voluntary.

What can go wrong with swallowing, especially in the elderly

A couple of changes which happen with aging make this phase of processing food more of a challenge. Taste sensation decreases, and older people seem to need more olfactory and taste bud prodding, so will empty the saltshaker a bit quicker.[1] With an ever-diminishing number of teeth, older folk have to chomp down on their food a greater number of times to prepare it for swallowing. Chewing muscles also get weaker. Dysphagia, or difficulty with swallowing, can occur in the initial voluntary phase of swallowing. A demented person, for example, may squirrel away food in his cheeks instead of initiating the first voluntary phase of swallowing.

Consequences of neurologic damage, such as cerebrovascular accidents/aspiration

Mr. Del had had a bad stroke. When feeding was attempted, he would choke, and rarely, food would exit through his nose. His issue was that the stroke had damaged his ability to protect his airway during the transfer of his food from the pharynx to the esophagus. His problem was recognized early, and had it not been he might have developed "aspiration pneumonia" because some of the food that took the wrong tube, i.e. went into the trachea instead of the esophagus, would become a focus for infection in the lung. Mr. Del would have to be fed in a different way, perhaps by a food tube in his stomach or small intestine or by his veins till his swallowing apparatus improved (19) (Geriatric Review syllabus, 9th edition, Chapter 30, PP 270-273, Colleen Christmas, MD)

Hiatal hernia and gastroesophageal reflux

Now we come to the esophagus, whose name, translated from the Greek, means gullet. It is a 10-inch tube composed of fibrous tissue and muscle, and its contractions push food down to the stomach. Its course wends posterior to the trachea or windpipe, behind the heart and through the diaphragm, which is that big muscle that separates the thorax from the abdominal cavity. A sphincter or valve separates the esophagus from the stomach. If that valve is lax, and doesn't close well, stomach contents can go up the esophagus and this gastroesophageal reflux can cause an acidic taste in the mouth, and even spill over into the trachea and bronchi. In those rare cases where the valve doesn't open properly, esophageal backup can occur. Both events can cause pain so severe that it sometimes can be confused with a heart attack

Poor salivary flow

Mrs T was approaching eighty when she developed a mild case of pneumonia. Her doctor, aware of her many proven and unproven allergies to medications, put her on a drug called tetracycline. This antibiotic, not too much used anymore because its spinnoffs are much better tolerated, is still a good drug for special circumstances. Mrs T had been having trouble with dry and sticky foods and usually washed them down with water. Her salivary flow was not as ample as it had been when she was young. However, she was tired after picking her medications up at the pharmacy, didn't bother to get water to facilitate swallowing the large tetracycline pill, and pretty quickly realized the medication had gotten lodged in her esophagus. Water after the fact didn't eliminate the problem, but a trip to the emergency room did. Salivary flow is reduced with aging, especially from the parotid gland, and many of the medications used for other problems can also diminish salivary flow. Dry mouth is a common complaint among seniors. Sometimes liquid medications become a better choice when available, and poor salivary flow, which can also have an effect on tooth health, may contribute to poor nutrition as well as swallowing difficulties.

Cancers and other issues

Unfortunately, cancers increase with aging and a decline in the function of the immune system. Esophageal cancer can be associated with cellular changes in the esophagus, with previous ingestion of caustic agents and with unknown factors. Persons with alcoholism or a history of cirrhosis of the liver from other causes can develop esophageal varices, which are essentially swollen veins that are prone to rupture and cause severe or life threatening bleeding.

THE STOMACH, NOT JUST A FOOD CONTAINER

The next stop for food is the stomach, which is blamed for every malady south of the chest. The stomach with its acid pH is more than just a container, and plays a big role in the further digestion of foods, which are composed of proteins, carbohydrates and fats, as almost everyone knows. The stomach's function is complementary to that of the small intestine, the major area of food absorption. Protein absorption, for example, starts when gastric pepsins are released, and the breakdown product, amino acid, help in the release of another substance called cholecystokinin, which in turn promotes the release of pancreatic enzymes into the small intestine. Carbohydrates and dietary starches in turn are broken down by the pancreatic enzyme amylase, which is also present in saliva. Fat absorption is also complex, and starts with emulsification, wherein fat droplets, which as everyone is aware are not soluble in water, are mechanically broken down to droplets coated with phospholipids in the stomach and elsewhere. Pancreatic lipase, secretin, and bile acids all play a role in regulating absorption and promote pH changes optimal for fat absorption. If all this sounds complex, we don't even know "the whole of it". New gastrointestinal hormones, neuronal pathways and a deeper appreciation for the friendly and unfriendly microbes that dwell mostly in the colon but elsewhere also have stimulated a blossoming of ongoing research into both the brain-gut connection and also into the roles these play in obesity, health and disease.

Things that can go wrong

Ulcers and gastritis

The first person to have his infection treated was the father of the family, whose stomach had been burning for a while, especially in the early morning or if he missed meals . Then the mother mentioned a similar pain in the upper part of her abdomen, and had a bit of anemia too. Finally, the whole family was brought into have their stools tested for a bacterium that had just been "discovered" in 1982! The family was duely treated with antibiotics and symptoms resolved. Our villain, a bacterium called Helicobacter pylori, is responsible for a large percentage of gastritis and ulcers....but it also is associated with stomach cancer. Eliminating it from the stomach, where it likes to snuggle down into the lining, cuts the risk of stomach cancer by about 2/3. Like so many viruses, bacteria, parasites and other unwelcome inhabitants of our mortal coils, this little bacterium is seen more often in persons from underdeveloped countries and is actually quite common in such areas of the world. For seniors from risk areas, who may not have had access to medical care in their native land, vigilance for this and many other types of infection is always prudent.

Lack of intrinsic factor

This story, recalled from a parasitology lecture in medical school, involves a special religious meal, a fish and anemia. During Passover, a very important Jewish feast representing God's sparing of Jewish firstborn males before the flight out of Egypt (Bible), gefilte fish is a traditional celebratory dish. This treat consists of cakes or balls made from deboned pounded white fish which may inadvertently contain a larval (immature) form of the fish tapeworm, Diphyllobothrium latum. Infected fish were, a century ago, usually imported from the Great Lakes to New York. Jewish grandmothers who were the usual preparers of this food, would taste it at different stages of boiling, using their culinary experience to judge whether it was cooked enough. They also inadvertently ingested the larvae. Unfortunately, if they ingested a large enough inoculum, or number of larvae, the tapeworms would happily grow and develop in their intestines. Absorption of vitamin B12, essential for red blood cell production, is a two step process. Intrinsic factor, produced in the stomach, is needed for the absorption which actually takes place in the small intestine. With a heavy infestation of fish tapeworms, this absorption was impeded, red cells could not be appropriately manufactured in the absence of B12, anemia developed, and even worse, B12 deficiency could also affect the nervous system!

B12 deficiency is not only attributable to fish. If the parietal cells in the stomach don't produce enough intrinsic factor, if these special cells are destroyed by inappropriate targeting by antibodies, if the small intestine is overgrown with bacteria, like weeds in a garden, or if the small intestine doesn't have the capacity to absorb the intrinsic factor-B12 combo, anemia and even dementia or psychosis may occur.

MR. M was 86 and his wife had died several years before. He lived a reclusive life in a second story apartment as a tea and toast senior. Dairy and meat were not on his diet, because his refrigerator had gone on the fritz a long while ago and his microwave was his only electronic kitchen friend. He did use alcohol, couldn't say how much, but it eased the pain and boredom of his existence. Not a guy to go to the doctor, his complaints of numbness in his feet went uninvestigated. Then he developed ataxia and his balance became a problem. Finally, his memory started slipping away. At this point, a nephew brought him to medical care, but not too much could be done. (Megaloblastic anemias, Bernard M. Babior and H. Franklyn Bunn in Harrison's Principles of Internal Medicine, Thirteenth edition, McGrw Hlii inc, 1994)

One of the screening tests for dementia is actually a blood exam for vitamins B12 and folate. However, any senior with a new gait disorder or other neurologic finding lacking other explanation, or with anemia where the red blood cells are larger than normal, will probably buy himself an investigation. Many seniors, as they age in place, don't have the energy, resources or will to create for themselves the kind of diet that would insure the presence of those vital vitamins so necessary for cellular metabolism. They may also not have the teeth to chew the meat, vegetables and fruits packed with those vitamins and minerals.

A very strong-headed little old lady with very disabling arthritis came for her first, and as it happened, last appointment at a clinic devoted to senior health. She had been taking a lot of over the counter Ibuprofen for her joint pain, and was developing a bit of stomach pain from popping it many times a day. She was, of course, told to stop, and given information on alternative treatments. She left in a huff, angry that her new physician didn't understand that no other remedies had given her the pain relief that lots of ibuprofen did. This class of drugs, of which there are several brands on the market, are highly associated with bleeding ulcers.

After her initial appointment, the clinic attempted to contact the little old lady several times by phone and letter, but no reply was forthcoming, at least not until one day almost a year later, when a policeman contacted the clinic about it's "patient". Our little old lady was found dead in her secluded apartment, possibly having bled from a stomach ulcer caused by overuse of a nonsteroidal medication, which could have led to other complications like shock or a vascular death like a heart attack partially caused by poor oxygen delivery to the heart muscle from anemia. We'll never know.

There are many medications which can be over-the-counter, and fairly harmless to younger patients, but devastating to elderly persons with little stamina. Another dangerous group of medications includes the proton pump inhibitors of which some brands do not require a prescription. Many people use these for indigestion/acid reflux and used briefly, they are helpful along with change in diet and other measures. However, these medications can predispose to pneumonia and to intestinal infection by reducing the stomach's function in fighting off bacteria.

Because there are so many medicines affecting the function, not just of the stomach but of the whole gastrointestinal tract, getting a history of every medication a person takes can be very important. Every medication and yes, herbs too, can have both good and bad effects. The elderly, with decreasing physiologic reserves, are especially vulnerable to side effects. For this reason, special attention is paid to all medications taken by older folk.

THE SMALL INTESTINE and ITS CRITICAL ROLE IN FOOD ABSORPTION

What the small intestine does

The small intestine is functionally divided into three parts. The duodenum is a 10 inch long somewhat "c" shaped tube extending from the pyloris, or opening from the stomach into the duodenum, to the jejunum. Its fame rests on being the site into which both the common bile duct and the pancreatic duct empty. These ducts carry enzymes which play a crucial role in digestion. It is also noteworthy for being the site at which peptic ulcers can develop.

The jejunum comes next. It is longer that the average pro-basketball player is tall by about a foot, and its lining contains mountains and valleys of cells critical for the proper absorption of nutrients. This "crinkled design "of projections called villi vastly increases its absorption surface.

The ileum is the last and longest part of the small intestine, and the site where vitamin B12 is absorbed. It empties into the large intestine through the ileocecal valve. This is also adjacent to where that problematic little tube called the appendix, dangles down.

The sections of the small intestine have many features in common besides being where almost all food absorption occurs. The peritoneum, an double apron of peritoneal tissue containing blood vessels, nerves, fat and lymphatics, attaches onto one side of the small intestines anchoring them to the back wall of the abdomen. The small intestine, besides being an absorptive surface, is also a muscular structure, pushing the food along to be absorbed, and the refuse to be delivered to the large intestine.

Let's follow our food through the small intestine. First, the fat marbling our steak. Already the lingual (mouth) lipase and the gastric lipase have created a lipid emulsion that upon entering the duodenum is further broken down by pancreatic lipase and colipase. Secretin mixed in with bile salts and fat-soluble vitamins form aggregates called micelles. These then go to and are absorbed into cells called enterocytes. In the enterocytes, a variety of fatty structures are packaged into aggregates known as chylomicrons, transported to the intestinal lymphatics and enter the general circulation. Meanwhile the bile salts themselves escape absorption, travel on to the end of the ileum and are reabsorbed there and trundled back to the liver for reuse. If this complicated series of interactions doesn't work perfectly, and fats are not absorbed at their proper locations, malabsorption and fatty diarrhea can occur.

Carbohydrate absorption is a little more clear-cut. Carbohydrate containing foods, like the milk-sugar ibn coffee, and are broken down by enzymes, mostly disaccharidases, and are absorbed. The process is actually a bit more complex depending on the sugars and starches being absorbed but not as complex as fat absorption.

Ms G was bloated, gassy and had diarrhea whenever she tried to eat ice cream, cheese, or milk. Her mother had become lactose intolerant too, as she grew older. The problem was easily solved. Mrs. G either used lactose free milk or she ingested the enzyme lactase before indulging in bovine created products. Lactase is a very important intestinal brush border (absorbing area) enzyme whose absence affects billions of people worldwide. These people usually lose their supply of lactase sometime after weaning age. Luckily, products containing lactase are on the market, or the enzyme can be supplied in pill form.

But the protein in the steak itself is a challenge. Here goes. Stomach pepsins like a low ph, but their ability to digest protein is impacted by gastric motility (contraction), the acidity of the stomach and what other foods are also in the stomach at the same time. Then cholecystokinin produced in the small intestine and other proteinases get together in the duodenum to break proteins down into their component amino acids. (enterokinase converts trypsinogen to trypsin that then activates to pancreatic proteases) These amino acids then get absorbed at the brush border with a little help from absorbing cells.

Most vitamins and minerals except B12 are absorbed in the first part of the small intestine. This fact is important for persons having a Roux en Y surgery for weight reduction. They may not absorb these vital vitamins and minerals well. (Joel.B, Mason, MD: Mechanisms of nutrient absorption and malabsorption, Up To Date, 2018 updated 10/10/2017)

The liver

Food that has been absorbed from the small intestine after processing, and ingested drugs, minerals and vitamins, travel through the portal vein to the liver. The liver is the body's factory. It further processes the products of digestion coming from the intestine via the portal vein,, detoxifies drugs and toxins, makes proteins, lipids and hormones, including clotting factors, and plays a part, as does the spleen, in cleaning the blood of harmful particles, like bacteria. It also makes bile. After the now highly processed and broken down food is worked on by the liver, it exits along with the other above liver products via the hepatic vein to the inferior vena cava and thence through the heart to be carried to hungry cells looking for energy.

What can go wrong with the small intestine: malabsorption

One case report told of a six-month-old baby who had been thriving on its mother's milk. Then came the time to introduce solids, so mother started cereals. Suddenly, things went south for this baby. Her growth, once robust, became very sluggish. Her astute pediatrician made the diagnosis, after testing, of celiac disease, a problem with absorption of gluten, a protein found in wheat. Celiac disease can occur at any age and changes the structure and function of the small intestine resulting in malabsorption, or failure of the above complicated processes in the small intestine to accomplish their job of getting the food we eat into our cells. There are many other causes of malabsorption which can cause serious damage to the health of seniors. Bacteria hang out in the colon. They should not hang out in huge numbers in the small intestine, for instance, and interfere with absorption of food products. Some people don't have the required enzymes to digest sugars and starches. Some others have had surgery on their small intestines, reducing the surface area of the bowel needed for absorption. Regional enteritis and other "autoimmune "problems also destroy absorptive cells. Some problems, like cystic fibrosis, are genetic and present from birth. Others are more subtle and can occur later, putting frail seniors at risk. But perhaps the problem we will have to deal with most often is weight reduction surgery.

It is not unheard of for seniors who have had multiple operations years ago, and who may be a bit forgetful, to fail to give a history of all their many surgeries. Most health care professionals make up for this problem during the physical exam, by querying patients on unexplained surgical scars and their origins. Such was the case with Mabel. At 66, she had had surgery on just about everything which could be safely removed: her uterus, ovaries, gall bladder, appendix. The surgeries were done long ago, at different hospitals, by different surgeons, for reasons Mabel wasn't very clear on. Getting the records would have been impossible. However, her provider was concerned about some of her abnormal lab tests. Her vitamin B12 was low, possibly contributing to her forgetfulness. Her blood showed an iron deficiency anemia. Medicine often involves detective work, which is maybe why the author of the Sherlock Holmes stories was a physician. At any rate, one other unmentioned surgery could have explained the lab findings. Turns out Mabel did have an operation called roux-en-Y, for her obesity a couple of decades prior. In this weight loss surgery, the stomach is attached to the second part of the small intestine, the jejunum, and in the process, some of the cells which absorb iron and vitamin B12, among other things, are bypassed, so these essential nutrients are not available in sufficient amounts to make red blood cells and help other body organs like the nervous system.

With more and more bypass surgeries to reduce weight being done due to our worldwide obesity epidemic, up to half of them bypassing areas of the small intestine where vitamins, minerals and other nutrients are taken into the body, information about past surgeries will be needed about older folk with symptoms like forgetfulness, falls, fainting.

Ms. T, in her early 60's, wasn't the best of historians. She had diabetes, anxiety, and a bunch of other medical and social diagnoses. Complaints changed every medical appointment. However, one complaint which remained at every visit was her diarrhea. It affected her truncated social life because she had to scope out the toileting facilities wherever she went. Sometimes the problem was bad, sometimes better. It took a year, and a lot of angst, but Ms. T and her partner finally came up with a suggestion. Would changing her diabetes medication, a drug called metformin, help slow down her diarrhea? A metformin holiday was arranged, and the diarrhea stopped, but Ms. T's blood sugar shot way up. Cautiously a lower dose of metformin was reintroduced, and finally a dose which controlled the sugar, and also caused a bowel frequency and consistency which was tolerable, was reached. That and a bit of self-control around the dinner table achieved a satisfactory outcome.

The Colon, Home for Billions, if not Trillions of Bacteria

Structure and Function of the Colon and Appendix

The colon is a tube ascending from your right lower abdomen up to your right upper abdomen where it makes a sharp left turn at the hepatic, or liver flexure, becoming the transverse colon, proceeding to your left upper abdomen, making a turn called the splenic (spleen) flexure then descending downward to your left lower abdomen. There an extension called the sigmoid, "s" shaped, stores feces for the rectum which goes down to your anus releasing stool at appropriate times. The first part of the colon, called the cecum, from which hangs the appendix, is separated from the small intestine by a valve called the ileocecal valve. The job of the colon is to rescue unabsorbed nutrients, wring the water out of the refuse of your digested food and create feces (stool) to be eliminated as waste. Peristalsis is the name of the muscular action of the colon and other parts of the gastrointestinal tract that propels food and feces forward.

The gut, especially the colon, also houses untold numbers of bacteria who are mostly our friends and make vitamin K, thereby preventing us from bleeding to death from a cut. Our gut bacteria come to live with us in a commensal union right after we are born. Gut bacteria in fact are the new frontier in gastrointestinal medicine. They help to maintain the health of the lining cells of the gut (enterocytes) and digest residual foodstuff in the colon, where they are in high concentration. A mucous barrier protects the colon itself from harm. It is estimated that about 3000 to 5000 or perhaps twice as many or more bacteria make their homes in the colon. Look for a lot more information coming to light in the future about the microbiome of the digestive tract, the hormones which connect the gastrointestinal tract with the brain, controlling appetite and other aspects of nutrition and function, and other aspects of this fascinating apparatus. (20) (Alexander Swidsinski, MD, Vera Loening-Baucke, MD, Up TO DATE, J. Thomas Lamont MD, section editor, and Deputy Editor, Shilpa Grover, MD, MPH, AGAF)

What Can Go Wrong

Dr. H was a college professor, attending a very important conference of educators, when his abdominal pain became so severe and colicky that he had to leave the meeting and seek care at his university's urgent care facility. Writhing in pain, he was seen immediately, and fortunately his pain abated long enough for an x-ray to be done. Turns out that this esteemed senior professor was severely constipated, or as some of his less enthusiastic students may have phrased it, "full of stool" except stool may not have been the technical term they would have used. The colicky nature of his pain, severe and then abating, gave a clue that with contractions of his colon muscles (peristalsis), the pressure and pain increased and when contractions were relaxed, pressure and pain decreased. Dr. H's problem was treatable with an enema and a program of colon care consisting of a change in diet to increased vegetables, fruits and other fiber containing substances, medications to speed up colon transit and regular fluid intake, largely water.

Occasionally, constipation becomes so severe that folk, especially the elderly, demented or cancer sufferers on high narcotics doses, need to be manually dissipated. This chore is usually given to medical students and is most distasteful, but also painful for the patient.

Fecal Incontinence

This very disturbing problem affected Mrs. G and prevented her from socializing with her friends. She' had damage to her anal sphincter during childbirth many years before and over the past year had a difficult time controlling flatus. Now she was experiencing passage of small amounts of watery stool. Defecation is a complex process involving the function of two sphincters, the ability to sense stool needing to e evacuated, voluntary relaxation of the lower (external) sphincter, the consistency of the stool and the whole process is worsened by prior injury to the sphincter, such as a difficult childbirth or hemorrhoidal surgery run amok. Dementia, developmental delay and the consistency of stool also come into play. A thorough history and physical, including a rectal and neurologic exam in Mrs G's case helped considerably with Mrs.G's problem. So did internal pressure recordings (anorectal manometry) .Nothing could be done about tear she had gotten when her son was born, but stool consistency and flatus were improved by taking her off her sugarless beverages and candy, and putting her on a lactose free diet . She had turned out to be significantly lactose intolerant. She was also put on psyllium seed to make her stool bulkier so liquid wouldn't leak through. These changes fortunately did wonders. She still would occasionally pass gas at inappropriate times, but her bottom worked well enough so she could resume her very important social encounters. The outcome is rarely as successful in demented patients, and often is a reason for placement. (21) (Anne E. Soumekh, MD and Philip O. Katz, MD, Chapter 52, Gastroenterology in Geriatric Review Syllibus, 9th Ed, AGS, Editors -in -Chief, Annette Medina-Walpole, MD, AGSF, et al, 2016)

Colon Cancer

Mr. T's story was a bit different from that of most persons with colon cancer. He didn't have any family history of the disease, but his relatives had lived in another country with little access to preventive medical care. He came in with his wife for well family care, and minimized the fact that he was passing maroon colored blood in his stool. He refused a colonoscopy, a procedure where under sedation, an instrument called a colonoscope is passed through the rectum and circled around to the cecum or beginnings of the colon, to pick up and pluck off polyps, or growths coming off the colon lining, before they became cancerous. If masses which could be cancerous are seen through the colonoscope, these are either biopsied or removed where possible. Mr T's wife and his doctor pleaded with him over several visits, but he remained implacable. One day about three months later he came back with a grin on his face and a healed surgical scar. His wife's badgering had gotten to him, he had his colonoscopy and then removal of what proved to be a malignant bleeding tumor in his colon, the cancer was fortunately fully resected, and he felt great and very proud of himself. This must be why men who are married live longer than those who are not!

Colon cancer is the second leading cause of cancer death in the US, and deaths can be greatly reduced by routine screening through specific stool tests or better still, scheduled colonoscopies beginning at age 50. Certain genetic problems or a family history of colon cancer may mandate earlier screening. Blood in the stool, a critical symptom, can be due to many other problems besides cancer but should always trigger a thorough investigation. It is important to note that since food ingested takes about 2-3 days arrive at the anus, blood from the stomach will probably make stools look black whereas blood from the rectum tum will be bright red, and blood from elsewhere will be intermediate in color depending upon where it originated. Certain substances like iron tablets and Pepto-Bismol will also turn stools black.

Bleeding-causes most common in the elderly

In fact, the list of circumstances that cause bleeding in the elderly is very long. For example, blood vessels in the gut can become tortuous and bleed (angiodysplasia), diverticula, largely in the colon can become infected and bleed, infections with a nasty bacterium called C. difficile can cause a rip-roaring infection in the colon with pain, bleeding and mucous, internal hemorrhoids in the rectum can bleed intermittently especially if a person is constipated...the list goes on and on. Blood in the stool tends to be more common in seniors, and perhaps our refined diets play a significant role in some of the causes.

Our knowledge of the gastrointestinal tract, its hormones, its connection with the brain, its resident bacteria, both villainous and protective, is growing by leaps and bounds. At this time, fecal transplant, though it sounds "gross", is saving lives in persons with severe, antibiotic-nonresponsive C. difficile colitis.

For or seniors, making the gut do its job may be the key to a long life.

CHAPTER 7

What the lung does and how it does it: Oxygen in, carbon dioxide out

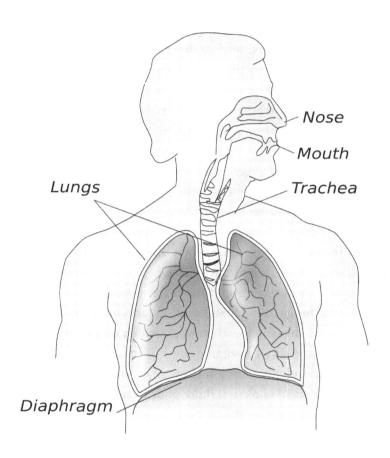

When you were a little fetus, snug inside your mother's fluid-filled uterus, you breathed the amniotic fluid in which you were immersed. Your lung tissue contributed to the making of that amniotic fluid. IN Fact, you started having sporadic and irregular breathing movements when you were just emerging from embryohood! Nothing during gestation happens in error, and the amniotic fluid which was made by and bathed your developing lungs helped your respiratory system and other parts of you to grow normally.(22) (Human Embryology, Organogenesis, module 18, online course in embryology for medical students, Universities of Fribourg, Lausanne and Bern (Switzerland)with support of the Swiss Virtual campus)

Which brings us to the question of how our lungs work after we emerge from the uterus.

Our lungs function a bit like green plants and trees...but in reverse. Leaves, for example, need carbon dioxide, and in the process, liberate the oxygen needed in respiration and metabolism by members of the animal kingdom. Since we are interested in humans, let's start with the basic structure where the exchange of carbon dioxide for oxygen takes place. This structure is called the alveolus, and enables animals to get rid of carbon dioxide, a waste product of our cellular metabolism, which can subsequently be used by green plants. By extrapolation, healthy humans are estimated to have about 300 million alveoli. No one has ever counted them, as far as we know.

Alveoli are thin-walled sacs at the end of bronchioles where the oxygen-rich air you breathe in is exchanged by diffusion from the tiny blood vessels, or capillaries, in the alveolar wall for the carbon dioxide which is a product of the metabolism of the cells in your body. Oxygen in, carbon dioxide out! The pulmonary arteries carry the carbon dioxide laden blood from the right side of the heart, to the alveoli. Obviously, the alveoli have delicate structures and are kept expanded by the action of proteins called surfactants, so they don't collapse.

How does air get from the nose to the alveoli? In the nose, hairs filter out contaminants. Blood vessels in the lining of the nose are very close to the nasal surface and help to warm the cold air which you breathe in on a winter's day. The rich blood vessel lining of the nose makes it easy to get nosebleeds, especially if nasal allergies make people rub and pick at the hardened mucous in their nostrils.

The air, containing about 21% oxygen, then traverses the nasopharynx, and pharynx. The pharynx or back of the throat, is the area where the openings at the end of both the nasal space and the mouth converge. The lower section of the pharynx opens into the esophagus or food tube and the trachea or windpipe. Attached to the trachea (windpipe) the epiglottis flaps over the esophagus to allow air to enter the trachea when one is breathing. From thence, the air goes to the bronchi, which like the branches of a tree, divide successively into bronchioles which get smaller and smaller in diameter until terminating in the alveoli.

How does air get into the lungs in the first place? The mechanics of breathing involve two sets of muscles, the diaphragm and the intercostal muscles, which when they contract, create negative pressure in the chest (thoracic cavity), dragging air in. The chest cavity is lined by a slippery membrane called the pleura, and the two lungs are also lined with slippery membranes, and these, lubricated by a small quantity of pleural fluid, glide over each other, permitting the virtually effortless creation of the negative pressure that allows air to rush into the lungs when we breathe in.

The lungs in maturity: what changes take place with normal aging

At age 69, Mr. P, an agricultural gentleman who had already survived a lung fungus and a goring by a noncompliant tractor, had a lifechanging event. He developed severe indigestion that just wouldn't go away. The "indigestion" stemmed from his heart problems. Nauseous and weak, the once massively muscled man allowed himself to be taken to the hospital, where coronary stents were placed, saving his life. On that day, he decided never to smoke again. However, his determination to lead a healthy life didn't extend to other aspects of his lifestyle, like eating prudently, exercising, visiting his cardiologist regularly and not running out of his medications. So one cold day about three years after his sentinel heart attack, he was pushed in his wheelchair into an urgent care clinic and gave a history of worsening breathing.

Since his retirement, and fueled by his heart attack phobia, he had become very sedentary. The more he didn't exercise, the more he had filled his time with eating. Now walking from the living room to the bathroom was a struggle. But that of course was not the proximate cause of his very real distress. He had picked up one of the bugs circulating in his community that December. He got pneumonia. His pneumonia put a big strain on his heart. His heart failed. He got swollen all over because his heart couldn't pump well enough to let the kidneys get rid of the excess fluid in his body. Without his medications…he had run out a while back, remember… his blood pressure climbed higher, putting a further strain on his heart. The oxygen in his blood plummeted further. His new health care provider, meeting him for the first time, took one long look and listen, hooked him up to oxygen, and immediately called the paramedics. A clinic was not the place for this man. He belonged in a tertiary care hospital, with a fleet of cardiologists, pulmonologists and intensivists.

Contrast him with another gent in his sixties. Same scenario, except this second man was a businessman. He took his heart attack very seriously, became an ovovegetarian with a smattering of chicken now and then, got a gym membership which he used daily, lost most of his paunch, and improved his sex life in the process. (He and his wife already had six children, so it was a good thing she was postmenopausal. Sending kids to college when one was in one's eighties would be difficult!)

Which brings up the question of what does happen to the lungs as we age, hooked in tandem to the heart as they are, and how many changes are somewhat under our control?

First let's talk about the alveoli, those air sacs where oxygen and carbon dioxide exchange actually take place. About one third of the surface area where gas exchange occurs is lost over a lifetime. Loss of elastic tissue means exhalation may be decreased, leading to lung hyperinflation when one is exercising maximally. Those little air sacks where carbon dioxide is actually exchanged for fresh new oxygen can coalesce, or fuse together, reducing the surface area so necessary for the actual carbon dioxide-oxygen exchange! This is probably only an issue for Master athletes, those older individuals who compete actively in Olympic types of events. What is an issue for the average Joe and Josephine is the fact that carbon dioxide diffusion capacity decreases approximately 5% a decade. That means when you are in your eighties, you experience a decrease of about 30% in your ability to quickly get rid of the carbon dioxide waste your body's cells have produced in exchange for fresh oxygen.

Decreases in air exchange apparently didn't bother Hidekichi Miyazaki, born in 1910, when he ran a 100-meter race in 42.22 seconds, breaking his former record in the Kyoto Masters at age 105. There are Masters competitions all over the world, every year, age stratified. People, male and female, compete up to and beyond their 10th decade. They exemplify the fact that though changes do invariably occur, dedication to an active lifestyle can maximize function way beyond what is the norm for most folk.

But back to the lungs. Several other changes happen, explaining why many old folks like Mrs. G do not want to live in a second or third story apartment. The lungs hyperinflate, due to the above-mentioned loss of elasticity, and it becomes more difficult to inhale oxygen needed for the exertion of climbing up several flights of stairs. Some alveolar sacs lose their blood supply, so they become "dead space" taking up lung but unable to contribute in the vital air exchange activity that is the whole purpose for our lungs' existence! What does all this mean? Less oxygen for all the little cells on our aging bodies. Fortunately the aging lung can still get rid of carbon dioxide…..unless lung disease intervenes.

Older adults are at especial risk in the low oxygen levels at altitude.

Now this isn't a big problem for Ms Daisy, a retired schoolteacher who lives on the first floor of her apartment building, spends her days viewing soap operas and morning discussion shows, and has her food delivered. But for Mr. M. it could be a huge problem in the days to come. After his coronary stent operation when he was in his fifties, he set his distant recovery goal on scaling Mount Everest. He is in his mid sixties now, and spends his abundant time as a quasi-mountaineer, going for long daily hikes up the local landscape, where baby mountains don't exceed an altitude of 6000 feet. A year or two ago, he made it to base camp on Mt. Everest at about 17.000 feet altitude. He's getting ready for another push this year and needs all the oxygen exchange capacity his older but well-trained lungs can give him.

An interesting article, written by an erudite columnist, Steven Hustad in SA Life in 2012, describes his conversation with a biologist at the University of Washington. This biologist studies, but apparently never published, the ages of Himylayan climbers. He found that risk of death accelerated quite a bit in climbers over age 60, but that one in 25 Everest climbers is over sixty! (23) (San Antonio Life, December 15, 2012)

The chest wall also stiffens and widens with aging, and the intercostal muscles between the ribs can create less chest expansion, forcing the abdominal muscles to take on more responsibility for creating the negative pressure that draws atmospheric oxygen into the lungs. Abdominal muscles do their best work when a senior is in a standing position. Efficiency declines when seated, even more so in the supine position. The diaphragm muscle also becomes less efficient, causing the work of breathing to increase by almost a third in some exercising folk. Although age related breathing changes decline less steeply in females than in males, reserve in the face of stress like pneumonia is still quite compromised in both sexes. If an older person does get pneumonia, he or she is less able to cough forcefully, clearing the air passages. Almost everyone is now aware that the Covid-19 virus is most lethal for the elderly with comorbid conditions.

This decline in the ability to clear air passages of mucous and germs brings back the saga of a lovely eighty something lady, the spinster aunt of a coworker. This lady had no one in the world except her very busy niece. When she developed a worsening "cold that turned into pneumonia", her niece brought her to the hospital, where she occupied an ICU bed for many days, taking several antibiotics, requiring higher oxygen delivery as she became more ill. Her pathetic little cough couldn't expectorate the bacteria-infested mucous secretions that her body was trying so desperately to get rid of. Her story did not have a happy ending in spite of the multiple interventions of her gaggle of pulmonologists (lung specialists).

But there is good news. A lung-friendly life includes not smoking anything, avoiding residence in such lung-unfriendly places at Beijing and Los Angeles, and especially religious fidelity to a lifelong exercise program, not to forget getting your vaccines against pertussis, pneumococcal pneumonia and other nasty bacteria. These strategies will keep your bellows functioning at maximal capacity for your age. (24) (Normal Aging, George E. Taffet, MD, Kenneth E. Schmader, MD, Section Editor and Lisa Kunins, MD, Deputy Editor, Up To Date, 2018)

Habits that harm the lung

Smoking, and that includes Marijuana

When Pedro (not his real name), an often homeless, middle-aged military veteran set adrift in a mountain community, gave up alcohol, he tried very hard to give up smoking too. He would come to his medical visits and boast of smoking only two cigarettes a day, or 5 cigarettes a day. When he failed to mention his cigarette statistics, his health care providers would assume that he was up to a pack or more a day. He was such a nice person, and tried so hard to please that it was painful to ask the nature and quantity of the pollutants he was inhaling. However, if Pedro were to have the long and happy life he deserved, helping him stop smoking became job number one.

Sally didn't much care if she were asked about her smoking habits. This sexagenarian lady, whose teeth had already exited her gums, would tell the interlocuter that she liked to smoke and that was that. Marijuana too, of course. When her habit's risk to her beloved grandchildren was brought up, her response was that she smoked outside. When this argument was countered with research showing that children whose relatives smoked outside still had levels of cotadyne, a byproduct of tobacco, in their blood, she changed the subject. A discussion of the cost of her habit (7 dollars a day by 7 days a week times 52 weeks a year x 40 years, a hefty down payment on a 4 bedroom house) was brushed off. Sally didn't remain a patient for very long.

Studies on e-cigarettes indicate great variation in composition. New data makes this a difficult subject to address simply, but most elderly persons using these products already have a significant tobacco history and need close attention to lung function and disease risk. A good deal of attention is also being given to the lung disease vaping is causing.

Most people consider lung cancer the biggest risk from smoking, but cardiovascular damage is a more frightening risk, and probably much more statistically significant. As an aside, an early menopause is another gift given to the habitual female smoker.

Living in Beijing, Los Angeles and other evil places

Pollution has existed even in ancient times. Many cities, notably Los Angeles, have cleaned up their air, but many other geographic areas still present air quality challenges. Persons who have spent their lives or portions thereof in such geographic or industrial areas are also at risk of lung disease as they age. Some cities even report air quality daily, so that those with lung diseases such as asthma and COPD can avoid exercising under conditions causing the inhalation of more pollutants. The National Institute of Health and researchers in other agencies have extensive data delineating the effects of high pollution on emergency room visits for respiratory illness. Longitudinal studies on geriatric effects of early life exposure to excessive pollution are, however, not robust. There is a good deal of interest among city planners in ways of eliminating vehicular pollution, a major contributor.

A seventy year old man presented himself to an urgent care facility for the first time, his tremendous girth dripping over the sides of his Big Boy wheelchair. Every time he had a paroxysm of coughing, he would stop breathing temporarily, scaring the nurses who couldn't figure out how to even get him out of his wheelchair should he need CPR. Before the paramedics arrived, and between coughing spells, he shared his extensive cardiac history and also another interesting fact: he had Farmer's Lung as a youth.

There are several occupations that put one's lungs at risk, and the residuals of these occupational diseases can have significant implications as people age. Farmer's lung and similar conditions are actually allergic or immune mediated reactions which attack the very small airways and the air sacks (alveoli) themselves.

Actually, there are a whole series of occupations that are associated with this "hypersensitivity pneumonitis", To name a few, there is coffee worker's lung, cheese washer's lung, woodworker's lung, even Japanese summer house hypersensitivity pneumonitis due to sensitivity to a fungus (Trichosporon cutaneum) found in bird droppings and possibly house dust. AS one ages, the damage due to these occupational disorders could be expected to compound normal aging changes. The treatment is, of course, mainly environmental control. Figuring out what specific trigger may be causing the lung's air exchange surfaces to "plug up" can be quite a challenge! (25) (Gary W.Hunninghake and Hal B. Richerson, Hypersensitivity Pneumonitis and Eosinophilic Pneumonitis, ppMcGraw-Hill1173-1176n in Harrison's Principles of Internal Medicine, 13th ed, T.R. Harrison et al)

Lung Conditions Commonly Seen in the Elderly

Pneumonia, Multiple Kinds

Pneumonia is the general term for a lung infection which causes the air sacks (alveoli) to fill with fluid and/or pus . The infection can happen in a part of a lung, a whole lung or both lungs. It is most common in very young children and in the elderly. It can begin insidiously perhaps with a cough which worsens, or it can make someone sick as a dog within hours. One of the reasons older folks are so much more susceptible than young adults have to do with the immune system and its components. These undergo aging, making seniors less able to fight off common bugs. Let's say an eighty-five-year-old man plays with his grandchildren over the Holidays. Their germ-laden little fingers find their way into his food and beverages. He is unaware of this. On one of those sticky little fingers is a whole colony of a nasty bacteria such as the pneumococcus. The individual bacterium love lung tissue, and divides about every 15-20 minutes. Doing the math, and barring interventions aborting this bug's fertility, an hour after inoculation, there are 16 pneumococcal offspring, by two hours, 256 and by 6 hours there are millions of these pesky organisms. Luckily, our bodies have a multifaceted defense system capable of repelling the unrestrained replication of these disease-causing bacteria.

Let's say a bacterium escape being sneezed out of the nose or coughed out. The air tubes (trachea, bronchi, bronchioles) have a mucous surface into which the bacterium might land, and specialized microscopic cilia or hairs, which act like little brooms, sweep bacteria and other unwanted particles upwards where they can be expectorated. Should a bacterium make it down to the air sack (alveolum), the body's immune cells working together with chemicals called cytokines identify the offending bacterium and facilitate its ingestion and subsequent killing by pus cells, or WBC's. The bloodstream of course sends in reinforcements as needed. This is a very simplified version of the lung's immune response. Please see the chapter on immunity for a more In depth overview of immune function.

As people age, their immune systems and body structure undergo changes which make pneumonia such a common problem that it is called "the old man's friend". Why? Because it is often the terminal event for very old folk. AS mentioned, the insults of a lifetime, like smoking and being exposed to allergens and pollution, "gang up" on people's lungs. The immune system can't do its job as well as it used to. Older folk have a weaker cough, can't generate the force to bring up those germs encased in mucous, which then sit in the lungs doing more harm. Fever is one of the body's defenses against bacteria and viruses, but older folk generally have a lower body temperature than younger folk and don't mount a febrile response as early or as well as is needed. Pus cells are slower to get to where the germs are. Often older people will become "septic" with pneumonia, because they can't cordon off bacteria well. These bacteria can break free and get into the blood stream. Then too, bacteria and viruses which normally affect very small babies whose immune defenses are still underdeveloped, come back in old age with a vengeance.

One bacterium which is a real problem in seniors is Mycobacterium tuberculosis which causes the disease TB.

One five-year-old child who was tested for tuberculosis developed a positive skin test, usually an indication of exposure to TB. His chest xray was normal, he had no signs of disease, but he did have the tuberculous bacillus somewhere in his body, walled off by his immune system so that he had no actual symptoms of disease. A thorough history revealed that he had visited his family in Central America several months before. His great grandmother had a cough but had not seen a physician about it. She believed It was a consequence of her age. Though it could not be proven, the likely scenario was that she had been exposed to someone with tuberculosis when she was a child, had "walled off" the bacterium, and had never had a problem until……….her immune system stated to decline and could no longer protect her against the mycobacterium tuberculosis she had lived with harmlessly for almost eighty years.

Back to her great grandson. We now had the tools to treat him and probably protect him from "reactivating" his tuberculosis germ when he gets to be 85. He was put on a drug called isoniazid. This drug and other similar medications have a good track record for squashing the "Latent TB reinfection cycle" seen in older people initially themselves infected in childhood.

Fungal and viral infections

It was the middle of the summer, but Mrs. T was very ill. She had a fever, cough, nasal stuffiness, bronchitis and pneumonia. Everything ached, her back, her joints, you name it. She sat in her hospital bed, a mystery to those of us caring for her until the pulmonologist came along and said he thought she had the flu. Tests proved him correct. The rest of us were baffled but impressed. Flu was a winter disease. Our prejudices prevented us from objectively looking at the symptoms this older lady had. Thank goodness for the pulmonologist, whose knowledge of the potential year-round presence of this virus, brought the medical team to the correct diagnosis. Fortunately, antiviral medications are often effective if used early: they prevent ongoing replication of the virus. Viruses, of course, are much much tinier than bacteria, are constructed quite differently, and replicate intercellularly. The reason the flu virus is so dangerous for older persons is often because of the damage it does to the respiratory tract, allowing other infectious agents to invade which otherwise couldn't do so.

Funguses are other agents that can cause pneumonia among other illnesses

For those who are curious, fungi have their own kingdom discrete from the animal and plant kingdoms. Some members of this exclusive coterie include mold, yeast and of course mushrooms/toadstools. These organisms can be breathed into the lungs. Most people never get ill from casual exposures. However, a subgroup of individuals, who may be geographically or immunologically vulnerable, will get bad disease from these organisms, which often gain bodily entrance through the lungs.

People who live in the San Joaquin Valley are especially vulnerable to developing a lung infection called Valley Fever, caused by a fungus whose handle is Coccidioides immitis. One can also inhale this organism when topsoil is disturbed and aerosolized anywhere from LA to Arizona and Northern Mexico. Soil and weather conditions must be just right for this fussy little dimorphic organism to propagate.

One mature and gracious lady, who lived in Los Angeles and had previously survived a bout of breast cancer, was found to have a nodule in her lung. Knowing that breast cancer likes to spread to the lung, her oncologist and lung surgeon were almost positive that a bunch of cells had broken away from her initial tumor before it was taken out and had found a new spot to grow in the lungs. This "metastasis" was biopsied. Imagine the lady's glee when the biopsy report came back that she had had Valley Fever! It seems that the lady's daughter had moved to Bakersfield, a city at the bottom of the San Joaquin Valley noted mainly for oilfields and country music. The patient had driven there once to see the grandkids but went from auto to house and back again in short course. Nonetheless, she had breathed in the fungus, managing to corral it into a small, pretty harmless nodule that probably never would have been discovered, let alone biopsied, were she not in the penumbra of her original cancer. Many regions of the world have their own species of fungal infections so asking a travel history is very important.

Viruses come in many different varieties, are roughly 1/100th the size of bacteria, and take over the innards of your living cells to replicate. Even plants have their own viruses. For example, the tobacco mosaic virus was discovered over a century ago. It was the first virus ever purified. It also can attack your tomato plants. Viruses are nucleic acids, either RNA or DNA, with a protein coat or capsid, and some have a lipid membrane or "envelope". Some famous viruses include Ebola, species of Coronavirus, and HIV. Viruses are also one of the more common causes of pneumonia.

Some viruses, like influenza, Covid-19 and respiratory syncytial virus, are especially virulent in young infants and again in older adults.

Hospital-acquired and nursing-home acquired pneumonias, both bacterial and viral, are real threats to the frail elderly . This is one reason why the influenza vaccine needs to be administered every year: there are several types of influenza viruses, which mutate with regularity. Vaccination is especially important in situations where the virus can spread from one disabled elderly person to another very quickly. Pneumococcal pneumonia, a bacterial pneumonia, is also a threat in such situations, and there are vaccines for the common types of pneumococcus bacteria most likely to invade the lungs. Of interest, when the pneumococcal vaccine was given to babies in the US, the rate of pneumococcal pneumonia in seniors dropped impressively. Little children were spreading the bacterium to their grandparents, and most likely are similarly spreading other diseases for which we don't have immunizations.

Other agents

Many older folk have difficulty clearing mucous due to the aforementioned mechanical changes in their chest walls and lungs, or due to reflux of stomach contents which can occasionally go down the wrong tube, or due to swallowing difficulties from strokes or other causes, leading to mouth and other bacteria getting into and multiplying in the lungs. These types of pneumonias are called aspiration pneumonias and may involve unusual species of bacteria.

Why pneumonia is the "old man's killer" : signs and symptoms of pneumonia in the elderly

One of the first symptoms of serious disease in very young babies is anorexia. The main task of a newborn is to eat and grow. This is why pediatricians automatically ask about appetite when the patient is very young. Unfortunately, symptoms and signs like fever, cough, congestion and even the ability to articulate distress may not be present in a timely fashion in the very old.

Mr. Y was ninety-one and lived with his daughter and her husband in a northern city during the winter. He really didn't seem ill at first. No fever, a bit off his feed, not quite as conversant as usual. The holidays were the center of everyone's attention, so his behavior wasn't really noticed much. He'd had the "sniffles" for a couple of days prior, but then so had everyone in the household. By the time he started to feel warm to the touch, and had become quite listless, his pneumonia was quite advanced. He died a few days later, despite hospitalization, antibiotics and appropriate care.

Very elderly patients have a delayed immune response to germs, which makes the extent of their illnesses difficult to estimate. They often don't mount a fever until late in the illness, and sometimes they can become hypothermic. Hypothermia is a lower-than-normal body temperature. It also sometimes happens in very sick newborns. Although a temperature of 99.5 would be perfectly normal for a one year old or a woman in the second half of a normal menstrual cycle (the temperature initially drops and then quickly rises with the production of the hormone progesterone after ovulation), 99.5 could be a raging fever in a centenarian. The reason is that as we age, our core body temperature drops a bit, and a normal temperature in a 75-year-old may be 97, not the expected 98.6. As mentioned earlier, the ability to produce a forceful cough is handicapped by changes of aging. Even reading a chest x-ray can be a challenge. Older people often have scarring on chest x-ray from earlier infections. The immune cells which migrate to the lungs to fight infection are more sluggish, so x-ray findings can lag behind the spread of the actual infection. Sometimes elderly folk with serious diseases like pneumonia will present with confusion or delirium, making it difficult to pinpoint the locus of infection. Then too, even with the best of antibiotics, the immune system may be too senescent to mount an effective fight against the pneumonia. Bacteria and viruses can break through these defenses into the blood stream and cause damage to other organs like the heart.

Asthma and COPD

As we age, we carry the dendritus of all the infections and insults our bodies have been through, coupled with the problems our genetics have imposed. Although smoking tobacco has decreased significantly over the past decade or two, marijuana and vaping have increased with yet to be appreciated lung consequences. The consequences of seniors' occupational and living choices also catch up.

Symptoms

Asthma and chronic obstructive pulmonary disease (COPD) can have similar clinical symptoms and are often intertwined causally. Lots of older people started smoking in the days before the Surgeon General's report warned of the many risks of smoking. They had difficulty giving up a very addictive and emotionally soothing habit when they became informed of the risks. Damage from tobacco (and presumably, other inhaled substances) can be partially but not completely reversed. Asthma, of course, is a genetic disease, often occurs with a viral or other infection or from exposure to allergens like cats or pollen. Both asthma and COPD involve narrowing of the bronchial air passages along with the production of inflammation and mucous. Cough, chronic or intermittent, is a feature of both. Asthma is more reversable after the stimulus is gone. Viruses and bacteria can both cause a worsening of COPD. Both asthma and COPD also are often treated with similar medications to open up narrowed breathing tubes and suppress the inflammation and mucous production. Both cause shortness of breath, the feeling of not being able to get enough air into the lungs, wheezing, and trouble sleeping at night when everyone's bronchi constrict a bit anyway.

Severity and its effects on quality of life

COPD, or a combination of COPD with asthma or other lung ailments, drains life insidiously and progressively. Asthmatic changes are often reversible, but this is not so much the case with

COPD. In fact, seeing ambulatory patients leave their hospital rooms to "go out for a smoke" just a few years ago was a phenomenon that made one realize that the reversibility of COPD is an emotional process as well as one of breaking a physical addiction. Eventually, anything that requires increased oxygen, like walking up a flight or two of stairs, and eventually, just walking to the bathroom, becomes very difficult. For those with far advanced COPD, devices that increase oxygen delivery become essential for everyday functioning. You often see these people tethered to wheelchairs and oxygen concentrators.

Mr D was a patient in a VA hospital. He was one of the first patients assigned to me when I was a medical student. He had fought in WW2, been introduced to cigarettes then, and continued the habit in civilian life. He died a lonely death, no relatives came to visit him, no-one seemed to care about his struggle to breathe. In those days, some of the tools and medications we now have for COPD weren't in use. WE all have patients we will never forget, and Mr D's struggle with COPD and the superimposed infection that ultimately killed him, will always haunt my memory.

Treatment in the elderly

Airflow limitation is the crux of treating asthma/COPD, and this can be measured but also declines just as a result of aging. Medications that enlarge the diameter of air tubes (bronchi) and reduce swelling and mucous production are helpful. Attention to conditions which may make the situation worse, like environmental allergies, can help too. As a last resort, seniors and others may have inability to get enough oxygen into their lungs due to their bronchial troubles (atmospheric oxygen content is only about 21% of inspired air, the remainder of the air we inhale being mostly nitrogen and a smattering of other gasses). Such patients can be given oxygen in much higher concentrations.

Cancers, nodules, and other things which shouldn't be in the lungs

Since all the blood in the body must pass through the lungs to pick up oxygen and get rid of carbon dioxide, cancers from other parts of the body often break off and travel to the lungs (the lymphatic system plays a big role here too). Even people who never indulged in tobacco, and especially those who did, can get primary lung cancer. Non-malignant scarring can be a response to long forgotten and overcome bouts of lung disease. Conditions like coal-miners lung are lifelong. Fluid can form in the pleural space, that space between the lining of the chest cavity and the lining of the lung. Emphysema is a condition where air sacks (alveoli) coalesce, and these can get so big that they "pop" or rupture. This rupture can create a pathway for atmospheric air to get into places it shouldn't, like the aforementioned pleural space. This air will eventually push the lung tissue aside. This series of events can kill if unattended to. Even food can get into the lungs by aspiration. All these happenings and more can compromise anyone's ability to breathe, but seniors are often already compromised through the aging changes they experience.

Keeping the elderly lung as healthy as possible

Healthy lungs start in infancy, if not before. Mothers who breast feed will protect their infants from lung infection. Vaccinating infants, children and adults against viruses and bacteria which can affect the lungs is a critical piece of lung health. This means that older folk deserve to have their grandchildren vaccinated appropriately. Choosing to live in a place with uncontaminated air can be helpful, but environmental allergies also need to be considered. (Current theory holds that perhaps exposure to allergens very early in life may be protective!) Some animals are more allergenic than others. People with a genetic risk for developing allergies may prefer not to fall in love with a kitten, or have their dogs sleep in their beds! People whose occupations expose them to particulate matter need to follow OSHA rules about using protective devices TO THE LETTER!

But if you are already 50 or 60, there are still opportunities! Stop smoking.... anything! Exercise, but start slow and work up, Keep your heart in good shape too. The lung, like other body parts, can heal itself, although maybe slowly and imperfectly.

CHAPTER 8

Why am I so thin skinned?

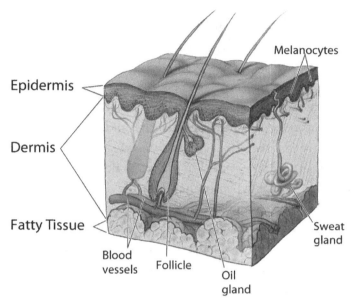

Epidermis

Dermis

Fatty Tissue

Melanocytes

Blood vessels

Follicle

Oil gland

Sweat gland

National Cancer Institute

Structure and function of the skin: Physiologic and immunologic changes over the years

Eleanor of Aquitaine was a Medieval lady of great intellectual prowess. She ruled the wealthy French provence of Aquitaine, was wife to two kings, Louis VII of France and then Henry II of England, gave birth to many children, of which one was Richard the Lionhearted, and another King John, the erstwhile villain in the tale of Robin Hood. She ruled England when Henry II was absent, went on the Second Crusade, and generally was one of the most remarkable women of her era. What is she remembered most for today? Her beauty!

Beauty is usually thought of as being a property of the skin, which is, of course, the largest organ in our bodies. It has, all told, an area of about twenty square feet. Of course, bones, muscles and other structures are the underpinnings of the skin and do deserve a bit of credit for one's appearance. But let's take a closer look at the skin itself,

Besides helping us to look attractive (or not!) the skin helps keep our bodies at a steady temperature by sweating and by shivering, depending upon whether we are getting overheated or chilled. Reptile skin lacks the necessary structures to regulate heat, forcing these generally disliked creatures to seek environmental modes of warming themselves, like sunning themselves on rocks.

The skin, although playing host to many commensurate bacteria, keeps bad bugs out. It also is the organ of touch, letting us know what is too hot or too cold to handle.

A brief review of skin structure permits a glimpse of how all these functions are accomplished. The outermost layer of our skin, called the epidermis, gives us our skin tone. Plump little babies are exceptionally endowed with good skin tone. The top of the epidermis waterproofs us. You will note that this top layer is much thicker on the soles of your feet, areas exposed to a lot of pressure and friction. The epidermis has the unique feature of producing a cascade of cells which grow upward from its more inward layers, and of sloughing the outermost cells as the newer cells grow upward to replace them.

Below the epidermis is the dermis, where the action happens. Its top layer (papillary layer) contains nourishing blood vessels and nerve endings and has a wavy surface that fits into the base of the epidermis like the pieces of a jigsaw puzzle. These surface projections are where blood vessels and nerve endings congregate. The blood vessels here, of course, nourish that top epidermal layer. Lipids to keep the epidermis moist and pliable, also generate here. With aging, this wavy interface flattens, making it easier for shearing to occur, and this change in structure can cause easy bleeding at the interface between dermis and the now thinned epidermis. The reduction in lipid production and a concomitant loss of skin glands makes geriatric skin dry and itchy. This problem occurs especially in winter when moisture in the air is reduced, and in summer heat. Thinning of the top epidermal layer and a reduction in melanocytes, those cells which give our skin its color, also makes geriatric skin less resistant to the environment.

To illustrate, perhaps you have had an elderly grandmother or aunt who liked to garden, but who inevitably got red bloody splotches underneath the fragile, dry parchment-like skin on her forearms after a session of weed whacking.

Changes in melanocytes producing skin color

Or take the case of Mrs. J. Her flawless ebony skin enhanced her beauty. This and her excellent bone structure made her appear 10 or 15 years younger. Her daily exercise schedule kept her muscles and tendons strong and plump. However, gradually, as her epidermis inevitably thinned, and her melanocytes receded, her skin lost a bit of its ebony sheen and tended more towards coffee color. Fortunately, Mrs. J's inner strength and childlike enjoyment of the wonders she found in each new day remained and continued to be transmitted to everyone around her, no matter her skin changes.

The deeper layer of the dermis, called the reticular layer, is especially problematic as one ages. it contains collagenous and elastic fibers running predominately in one direction corresponding with the tension skin lines that become more prominent with the stretching of our movements. If you should ever need surgery on your skin, for example, if you require the removal of a troublesome cyst, your doctor will probably plan the incision he or she has to make to correspond with these tension lines and therefore minimize scar formation .

Thinning and loss of cells/ reduction in cellular immunity

Unfortunately, the elastin fiber network, so important for skin resiliency and health, begins to decline as early as one's thirties! Sweat glands in the skin decrease, making it difficult for older persons to cool themselves in very hot weather. The skin's immune function and the cells which facilitate the ability to fight invading organisms also wanes. Simple cuts, repaired promptly in young skin, can become life threatening in the very elderly patient.

That is what happened to 89-year-old Mrs. Z. She took a plastic trash bag out to her garbage container at the end of her driveway. A piece of a broken glass poked its way through the trash bag as she dragged the bag to her curb and cut her ankle superficially. When she was seen right after this minor laceration, it didn't even need stitches, so was only cleaned and bandaged lightly. Two days later, she presented with a rip-roaring infection. Outpatient antibiotics didn't help, the ankle became more swollen and redder, so poor Mrs. Z had to spend the better part of three days in the hospital getting intravenous antibiotics for a cut that a baby's skin would have healed practically overnight. And all for taking out the garbage!

Underneath the dermis is found connective tissue, fatty tissue and the superficial fascia, giving further contour to the skin. In some places, the skin undersurface is attached through connective tissue bands to underlying structures. In others, like some areas of the face and neck, the muscles themselves attach to the underbelly of the skin. If you have dimples, that phenomenon is at work. (26) (Textbook of Anatomy, Fourth ed, W. Henry Hollinshead, PhD and Cornelius Rosse, MD, D. Sc, Harper and Row, Publishers, Philadelphia, 1985, Chapter 10, pp 139-143)

Skin appendages: structure and changes with aging

A word about other important skin structures. Sweat glans come in several varieties. They regulate body temperature, and most open directly into the skin surface. However, those glands in the arm pits, the genital areas, and the breast nipples discharge into hair follicles, and give odor to sweat. They also enlarge at the time of puberty, a fact to which anyone who coaches teenage sports can attest. The sympathetic nervous system is intimately connected with the production of sweat. Earwax is also made by modified sweat glands, and in older persons, often becomes dry and impacted, reducing the ability to hear. Sometimes a good earwash can magically restore auditory function in a senior as it did for Mr J. The look of astonishment on his face as big plugs of orange-brown wax were flushed out of his ears was priceless. He could hear again!

Sebacious glands make an oily material that coats the hairs that emerge from hair follicles all over our skin. These glands can also open directly onto the skin, especially in the nose, eyelids, genital and nipple areas.

Then there is hair, a woman's "crowning glory" and the subject of everything from Broadway hits (ie, the musical from the 1960's) to fairy tales like Rapunzel. In this story, you may recall, a beautiful teen with a head of long hair was rescued from imprisonment in her locked tower by a prince who uses her tresses as a rope.

Hair follicles live in the dermis of the skin, and produce strands of tightly packed cornified cells called, of course, hair. On our bodies, hair follicles are associated with bundles of smooth muscles that can "make our hair stand on end" Hairs are constantly falling out and being replaced, and in early adult hood, becoming thicker and coarser in some places. Unfortunately, as we age, hairs thin, and follicles may atrophy completely. Loss of pigment, or whitening of hair, has somewhat of a genetic basis too.

Nails are also tightly packed cornified epithelial cells growing up from the nail bed which is fed by nerves and a blood supply. Nail growth is reduced by about 50% in older folk. Their yellowing color may also be unappealing.

The effect that normal aging has on the skin and its appendages then is profound. The changes induced by aging often are more problematic for light skinned folk and for women. Skin loses tissue, can't repair itself as well, has decreased resilience to trauma, a decreased ability to fight infection, and to regulate body temperature through sweating. It gets dry from decreased lubrication, leading to itchiness. Thin skin bruises easily. It changes color due to loss of melanocyte function, and its blood supply diminishes, with remaining blood vessels often undergoing constriction, causing a more sallow color. Additionally, hair thins or is lost, while also changing from the vibrant colors of youth as its pigment diminishes. Skin sensory perception also is reduced, more so in the lower extremities. A hidden problem is a loss of vitamin D. (27)(Up to Date, www up to date.com,Normal aging, George E. Taffel, MD, Section Editor, Kenneth E. Schmader, MD, Deputy Editor, Jane Givens, MD)

Vitamin D and the aging skin

Vitamin D has gotten a lot of well-deserved attention. In the epidermis, the ultraviolet rays in sunlight change a chemical called 7-dehydrocholesterol into previtamin D3 . AS the skin loses its supply of 7-dehydrocholesterol, and as older folk become more housebound, less vitamin D is made.

Vitamin D is more than a vitamin. It is very important for bone repair, for muscle health and plays an important role in the immune system. Some researchers even call it a "hormone" because of all it does.

Although vitamin D is especially important for postmenopausal women who have an increased risk of osteoporosis and fracture, it can be necessary for older men as well, though they lag a decade or so in the development of bone loss.

Mr P, for example had become addicted to television after his retirement at age 70, and had developed the usual consequences of a fatty paunch, weakened muscles and so forth. Although he lived in the mountains where the sun's rays were more penetrant, his vitamin D levels had fallen to very low levels. Spending more time in the sun probably would not do the trick for this gentleman, since his ability to produce vitamin D was restricted by his aging epidermis and his decreased kidney function, kidneys and liver also being important for production of vitamin D. He had to be treated with whopping doses of vitamin D and then placed on lifetime smaller doses!

Protecting aging skin

Wrinkles

Mrs. T's mother, a World War II bride from Japan, would not leave the house on a sunny day without her "parasol" or umbrella. She urged her daughters to do the same, but they considered her practice of sun avoidance an embarrassment. They were also of the generation which believed that a healthy tan was a key element of beauty, so would spend hours on weekends lying supine in the back yard, and later on the roofs of their college dorms, to soak up the sun's rays. Inevitably, wrinkles ensued, especially since both daughters took up smoking cigarettes in college.

Wrinkles are a combination of skin aging and exogenous damage. Frequent use of specific groups of facial muscles may accentuate furrows in certain areas. You yourself may have been told as a child not to frown so much!

Photoaging, or solar damage, certainly contributes to wrinkling, but so does smoking and the natural changes of aging wherein the epidermis thins and the wavy dermo-epidemal junction discussed above loses its undulations. Fibroblasts, those cells whose mission it is to repair skin, weaken. Importantly, elastin synthesis starts to diminish as early as one's thirties. Important large molecules in the dermal layer of the skin tasked with supporting cutaneous resilience and hydration fade too.

However, if one really wants to accelerate skin wrinkling, the best method is to smoke a lot. Mrs P was only 57, but it wasn't even necessary to take a tobacco history from her, or to appreciate the smell of smoke on her clothing. Her deeply furrowed face told the story of her almost lifelong 2 pack a day smoking history. Her lung exam completed the picture, demonstrating poor breath sounds and an occasional wheeze at rest. Smoking, of course, constricts blood vessels, which are the body's means of supplying nutrition, and damage repair to all organs including the skin! As an aside, Mrs P had probably spent over 150, 000 dollars in currant monetary terms, on her habit. Wisely invested, this wasted money would have kept her off the welfare rolls. Unfortunately, all she got for her monetary outlay was a bunch of wrinkles, damaged lungs and in her case, damaged coronary arteries and an early menopause!

Sun damage

Solar exposure also ages the skin, with perhaps the greatest damage being done in childhood. Persons with bad sunburns in youth are at increased risk of certain skin cancers as they age. Of note, the current generation of mature folk wasn't swathed in sun block when they were young as is a common practice nowadays. Even today, though, the need to reapply sun blockers every 2 hours, and when swimming, may not be on every parent's radar. However, solar damage is distinct from skin aging itself.

Although darker skinned people have some protection, that protection is not absolute, as Mrs G discovered on her Hawaiian honeymoon. A very dark skinned African American, she felt immune from sunburns, so she baked for many glorious relaxing hours in the wonderful Hawaiian sun. The result was a painful sunburn which marred the tail end of her otherwise wonderful new marriage. Now a mother, Mrs G made sure her kids were always protected from the sun. She carried the message to her friends who also thought their skin color provided invincibility.

There is a tradeoff in using solar protection. Vitamin D generation requires some sun exposure. The sun's rays are most powerful between 10 am and 2 pm. Total avoidance will reduce sun damage and the risk of skin cancer but may result in low levels of vitamin D. Elderly persons often require oral vitamin D2, and this is in fact recommended routinely in postmenopausal women.

Injury

AS the epidermis (outer skin layer) thins, the skin's blood supply is lessened, the immunologic Langerhan's and other cells in the skin diminish in quantity, and the junction between those two skin layers, the epidermis and the dermis, flattens. Older skin is very vulnerable to injury and infection and heals more slowly. Healing, itself, is a multistage process engineered by reparative cells in organized stages and dependent upon a healthy blood supply and good nutrition to get the materials and worker cells to the area of injury to do their job. Any condition that impairs blood flow to the skin, for example, the changes in blood vessel flow that often accompany aging, or prolonged pressure from not being mobile, can result in breakdown of the skin with resultant poorly healing ulcerations .(28)(Basic principles of wound healing, David G Armstrong, DPM, MD, PhD, Andrew J. Meyr, DPM, IN Up To Date, Russell, S Berman, MD et al, Section editors, WWW uptodate.com,2019)

Mrs J age 92, unfortunately suffered a laceration over her left shin, an area of the body where the skin and bony covering (periosteum) meet and where cushioning and capillary assistance from muscles and other tissue is not available. The tissue-thin skin was just too delicate to suture. Any attempt to place sutures would just have ripped open more skin. She ultimately had her torn skin held together with steristrips, which are like scotch tape for wounds. Infection was a big concern too.

Sometimes skin breakdown comes from inside and not from external forces like cuts or burns. Mr. T had poorly controlled diabetes and smoked his inactive days away. The blood supply to his feet dwindled, till his doctor couldn't even feel his pulses there. Moreover, he developed pain in his legs when he walked farther that his mailbox and had to sit and rest until the pain went away. So, he stopped walking and this made things worse. Eventually the arterial blood supply to his feet got so bad that he developed a sore on his toe that turned into an ulcer and that ate its way down to the bone. He wasn't alerted to this process because his bad diabetes had damaged the nerves in his feet. Pain signals weren't being sent appropriately to his brain. Furthermore, he never bothered to check his feet daily, as his doctor had enjoined him to do. The end result was an infected toe bone and an amputation. A similar process sometimes happens in persons suffering from a stroke or other severe immobility and unable to move about in bed. They can develop ulcers over bony prominences like the lower spine and pelvis called bed sores. These can erode down to bone and cause not just local, but sometimes systemic infection.

Burns are a big concern in the elderly.

Rashes and serious skin changes

Types of skin cancer

In general, cancers just don't pop out of nowhere. Cells and other parts of our immune system, including vitamin D, take down rogue cells before they can multiply and do damage. Exposure to "environmental carcinogens" is ongoing through life, so we need a vibrant immune defense not just against infectious agents like bacteria, fungi and viruses, but also against our own cells gone wild. Skin cancers are some of the more common types of cancer people develop as they get older and their immune systems also age and become less capable of destroying wayward cells.

What to look for

Mr. W, as a tow haired, pale white child in the 1950's, never used sun block, was raised on a farm and from early childhood ran around shirtless and hatless on sunny summer days. His first cancer appeared when he was in his fifties, and it was caught early. Thereafter, Mr. W insisted on yearly head to toe examinations of his skin. Several more skin malignancies popped up through the years. Knowing that the chances of developing skin cancers often ran in families, Mr. W was merciless in stalking his four sisters and brothers until the whole family got into the habit of yearly dermatologic exams. One sister also had recurrent problems, another brother detected a malignant melanoma, the most vicious type of skin cancer, early before it had a chance to spread.

There are three main types of primary skin cancers, and they can develop on sun exposed areas, and occasionally in more hidden spots.

Basal cell carcinomas are the least dangerous in that they tend to grow in place and rarely spread to other organs. They appear as pearly papules or "bumps" often bordered by a network of very fine blood vessels called telangectasias. They like to grow on-sun exposed areas like the face.

Squaemous cell cancers also like to appear on sun exposed areas and often grow on the lower lip or the ear. They are firm crusty growths that can ulcerate.

Malignant melanomas are the most feared of skin cancers. They do spread to internal organs. New treatments show promise, however. Melanomas have several features that make them stand out. They have irregular borders, that are said to resemble a "map of Maine". They have an irregular contour, with peaks and valleys. They can be skin colored but usually are dark and contain many different shades of brown or black cells within the same area. In other words, they are multicolored. Bleeding or ulceration are late findings. (29) (Arthur J. Sober, and Howard K Koh, Melanoma and other Pigmented Skin Lesions, Chapter 325, in Harrison's Principles of Internal Medicine, 13th ed, Kurt J. Isselbacher et al, editors, McGraw Hill, Inc, USA,1994)

Because of the many changes in skin color and texture that occur as people age and that are not cancers, skin issues need to be brought to the attention of a skin specialist if concerns exist. Concerns include a skin abnormality that is new or growing, one that is painful, bleeding or beginning to ulcerate, or that is in an unusual place, accompanied by fever or other symptoms. When concerned, check it out with a professional!

How skin cancers are thought to develop

Much research has intimated that bad sunburns in childhood may set the stage for the development of skin cancers in mature folk. Children growing up in the mid twentieth century often were not protected from the sun. Tanning and solar beams were considered healthy, and sun blockers were not commercially available as they are now. Even today, many parents are unaware that sun blockers need to be reapplied every two hours, especially if a child is sweating, and after water contact. Prime candidates for developing skin cancers are freckled fair, blond or redheaded folk, those with a family history of skin cancers, and especially those in their senior years. It is very important to remember, however, that even very dark-skinned persons can develop skin cancers and need protection. They too deserve evaluation of any concerning skin changes. Since sunlight is also important for making vitamin D, protection from excessive sun may involve paying close attention to vitamin D.

Treatment of precancer and cancers of the skin

If a precancer or skin cancer is found, many factors go into deciding on the best treatment. These include the type of precancer or cancer, the degree to which it has grown, whether it has burrowed into deep layers of skin, or even spread to internal structures, and the risk that it will reassert itself. Some precancers can be treated with topical medications or other local interventions, others will need extensive surgery, and still others may respond to the "big guns" used for cancers which have spread elsewhere in the body. Immunotherapy is the new kid on the block to treat cancers and many other maladies. It involves alterations in our complex immune systems to allow the extermination of malignant cells, but these alterations can sometimes cause collateral damage too. The most important issue, however, is early identification of potentially dangerous skin changes.

Shingles: The long life of the chicken pox virus hidden int the nerves and: how to recognize the rash

Mrs D was a joy to have as a patient. She was a poet and writer, was very intelligent and conversant with what was going on in the world, was unfailingly kind and interested in a good way in other people. She was eighty-three. One day, however, she was brought in by her niece and was in a state of confusion. There was a trail of very small blisters on a red base, some of which had run together and merged. This painful rash followed the course of her fourth right thoracic nerve right onto the section of skin (dermatome) to which that nerve gave sensation. Mrs D was in a great deal of pain, having had the rash for several days already. She was treated with an antiviral medication a bit late, since these drugs are decidedly more effective when used right away. Pain medications were added but were not too effective. The pain was so great that Mrs D's confusion and irritability continued for months. Then one day Mrs D returned, and amazingly, she was back to her cheerful, interesting self.

Mr S age 73 had a different course. He spoke Spanish and was hard of hearing. Translation failed to uncover the subtle specifics of his complaints. What was apparent was that he was having severe left sided chest pain. So, paramedics were called to the clinic and he was packed off to the emergency room to be worked up for a heart attack. In the process of the work-up, he was noticed to have the beginnings of a left chest rash, again in a "dermatome" distribution, with tiny blisters. The heart attack evaluation was normal. Mr S had shingles.

Although most children are now vaccinated against the chicken pox (varicella) virus shortly after their first birthday and again when they turn four, this vaccine schedule is relatively new. Persons in their senior years, and even people as young as their late thirties, got the disease and not the vaccine. Since it was known that chicken pox was a much worse disease in persons after adolescence, many mothers arranged in the days before vaccination was available to have "chicken pox parties" . Preschoolers were invited to play with a child having active chicken pox. Varicella is a very contagious disease, and the mothers hoped that by getting the disease early, their children would have a less serious infection and would develop immunity which would protect them in later life.

All well and good, but the varicella virus has a secret trick. It never goes away. It hides out in the dorsal ganglia of the spinal cord. The dorsal ganglia are nerve bundles adjacent to the spinal cord where nerves from the brain communicate with nerves that go to specific skin segments called dermatomes. For reasons unknown, the virus can become reactivated, travel down the nerve to the skin, and cause a blistery red based rash that actually contains the chicken pox virus in the blister fluid. This rash is called shingles, and can involve different dermatomes. Generally, pain precedes the appearance of the rash by up to 2-3 days, and in older folk the pain can be very severe, often described as burning. This is why it is sometimes thought to represent a heart attack or other catastrophic event. Interestingly, though, when younger persons get shingles, it is often painless or only mildly itchy.

Treatment and sequellae

Rapid detection and very early antiviral treatment are very important, but difficult unless the victim recognizes symptoms in the pain stage. About one third of folk will get shingles in their lifetimes, and it can be recurrent. The rash is characteristic which means that most medical personnel and even patients and their family members will recognize the rash.

When shingles is not treated immediately, and often even when it is, postherpetic neuralgia can cause severe and even disabling pain for months afterwards. This is why many physicians and other providers will give patients a medication to help with nerve pain (neuralgia)at the same time the antiviral medication is given.

Prevention and amelioration

There is now a potent vaccine which can prevent shingles. (The old vaccine was not very powerful). However, this new vaccine causes transient side effects in 9 out of 10 people and is not currently available in some places. It should be widely available very soon.

For those who are not protected by the new and potent vaccine, pain can be the most important aspect of care after specific antiviral treatment. Specific medications directed towards nerve pain are helpful but not often curative. It is important to remember that severe chronic pain can cause personality changes in seniors, but that the pain ultimately will go away,

Age spots, seborrheic dermatitis, black and blue marks and other curses of aging skin

Unfortunately, aging and genetics aren't the only reasons for skin changes. What people did in their younger days haunts their skins too. Sunbathing and smoking, two popular social activities for those who came of age in the 1960's and earlier, have cursed their now older protagonists with ungainly skin. Photoaging, which reflects the cumulative exposure to ultraviolate light. usually from the sun, sometimes from tanning salons, can ultimately cause many unwanted changes. These include age spots, patches of excess pigment or too little pigment, thin webs of fine tiny blood vessels known as telangectasias, skin loosenes, a sallow color and a leathery feel to the skin.

Perhaps you have seen on occasion a matriarch wearing bright colors, makeup so thick it was practically flaking off, vivid red lipstick, and off color eye shadow. This was the case when a group of paramedics climbed the narrow stairway to the vacation home of a 97-year-old widow lady complaining of chest palpitations and pain. Beside the bedstand was her picture as a flapper in the 1920's. In those days, she had been young, truly beautiful and apparently rich too. She held tight to that persona her whole life, to the extreme of making her paramedic rescuers wait while she finished applying her make-up.

On the other hand, there was Mr. M, a gnarled, lean retired farmer. He often did the heavy work in his fields shirtless, and now his back was thickly populated with ugly dark waxy warty, irregular patches and plaques, with a stuck-on appearance, up to 4 cm in length/width. These patches, when mature, could sometimes be peeled off, and underneath was pink baby-like skin. Mr M had seborrheic keratosis. Sometimes these fairly common skin findings can be difficult to differentiate from skin cancer, and need a biopsy, especially when they are very darkly pigmented. However, they are benign.

Skin changes that mean things are going wrong elsewhere in the body: yellow skin

Mr. X was a young senior, who came into clinic initially, leaning heavily on his walker, and without any medical records. He thought Truman was the president, got angry when corrected. He probably didn't need his medical records, since his diagnosis was very apparent from a precursory inspection of his skin and eyes. Both were yellow. The undersurfaces of his eyelids, however, showed good red color. He couldn't balance without the support of his walker.

Mr. X was jaundiced, implying either that his red blood cells were breaking apart or that his liver was failing. The rich color of his conjunctivae suggested that his red blood cells were OK. His lack of balance hinted at the neurologic consequences of excessive alcohol use. His confusion suggested that his liver was not processing toxic substances as it should. In short, one look and one question strongly suggested alcoholic cirrhosis. His girlfriend affirmed the diagnosis.

Most people with sallow skin are not cirrhotic. A sallow color can intimate the normal changes of advanced aging, it can represent skin color normal to the individual, can signify vascular disease with a poor blood flow to the skin, and in infants may even indicate an excessive intake of vitamin A! However, more abrupt changes in skin color do merit a search for a variety of diseases.

Nail changes

Nail changes can give clues in both young and older folk, to the presence of disease. Onychomycosis, a fungal infection of the nail plate, especially that of the great toe, causes thickening and color change. The nail frankly looks ugly! Although onychomycosis can happen at any age, it can cause pain and even ulceration if the sensation of pain is absent (peripheral neuropathy) Older folk have a higher frequency of obesity, diabetes, immunity problems and poor circulation when this nail problem is present. Nails in older people especially toenails, grow very slowly, so medications either by mouth or topically, take a long time to work and are not always effective!

Folk with so called "spoon nails" can have severe anemia. That was the cause in a woman living under very harsh social circumstances in a desert community. The cause turned out to be bleeding from her uterus. When an older person has severe anemia (low blood), determining the cause becomes critical. Naiil changes can alert health care personnel to serious medical conditions.

Nails that are clubbed, bluish and/or have a diminished angle between the nail growth plate and the skin of the thumb/finger may have heart/lung disease. Folks with pitted nails need to be checked for psoriasis and psoriatic arthritis. Unusual nail bed capillaries may indicate autoimmune disease. Pale nail beds can also signify mild to moderate anemia. Yellow nails may be just the result of aging itself.

Unexplained darkening of the skin

Mrs T was in her late forties. The mother of two children, she noted fatigue, nausea and weakness which progressed very slowly over the course of months. When she finally got to the hospital, her blood pressure was quite low, her skin darkened, and she hadn't the energy to even get up out of bed. Weight loss was significant. Changes had happened so slowly that the family had overlooked them, her husband taking over some of the household chores and the kids, who were older, pitching in. Not until Mrs T couldn't even get out of bed were her symptoms taken seriously. Though she was Hispanic, it was immediately evident to her doctor that her skin and even the inside of her mouth were much darker than her ethnic heritage would have allowed. Mrs T had Addison's disease, a problem with the function of her adrenal glands seated astride her kidneys. She was no longer producing much of a very essential hormone called cortisol. The story ends happily, with the exact problem being uncovered and Mrs T returning to full function.

Mrs J's skin color also was darkening slowly, but in her case, her ethnicity was northern European. She also had darkening of her skin, weight loss and elevated glucose. Sexual relations with her husband had become a burden. She chalked it up to her "change of life" because her symptoms started after her menstruation stopped with the onset of menopause. Family history revealed that her father had died of liver failure in his forties, chalked up to excess alcohol ingestion. However, she remembered him as pretty tanned. Mrs J had hemochromatosis, in which excess iron is absorbed and subsequently stored in organs like the liver, heart, joints, gonads etc. Women during their reproductive years, get rid of excess iron through menstruation. Therefore, symptoms are delayed in onset. Not so for men.

Odd vascular rashes

Mrs. W was disconcerted by little red polyp-like bumps popping out mainly on the skin of her upper chest. She first noticed them after her menopause but conceded a few may have been there earlier. These lesions are widened capillary tufts flowing into congested venules, are called cherry angiomas and are quite benign and usually quite small.

Mrs A had very nice legs. At least she had always been told that was so. Now at age sixty-something, and after birthing several children, she was developing a fine network of purplish venules on her legs accompanied by a coarser presence of varicose veins.

On the other hand, Mrs B had a fine network of very red threads of blood vessels radiating from a central punctum, called spider angiomas. She'd gotten a few with her pregnancy too. Her doctor told her to wean down on the estrogen replacement she had been taking for her menopausal symptoms

Vascular changes are common as persons age, can occur on the skin and elsewhere, and are usually benign. They are often associated with the increased tortuosity and changes of aging that occur in the blood vessels of the body .

Easy bruising

As the skin ages and thins, bruising related to very minor trauma increases. Persons on drugs like aspirin may also note increased bruisability. Mrs J noted that every time she gardened, she would get bruises and cuts from her roses and other thorny plants. They took a few days to clear up completely. She didn't care. Her gardening brought her too much pleasure and relaxation for a few forearm bruises to interfere with this hobby.

Again, light skinned seniors, and especially women, are more affected. Africans and African Americans, with their beautiful, more resilient skin, are significantly protected from this curse of the fair skinned individual.

Changes that come from cancers elsewhere

Several cancers can have cutaneous manifestations although they originate elsewhere. This is why any unusual, expanding, painful, bleeding or new skin lesion needs a look-see from the patient's health care provider!

Covid 19 skin problems

Our new friend, Covid`19 has been associated by dermatologists with a variety of skin rashes. Although the exact connection is uncertain. Hand foot and mouth disease, a self-limited viral illness usually seen in young children, and shingles occurring at an earlier than expected age are sometimes seen. These skin problems may just be coincidental with Covid, and luckily they are not serious.

CHAPTER 9

The Nervous System: Its Function and Anatomy

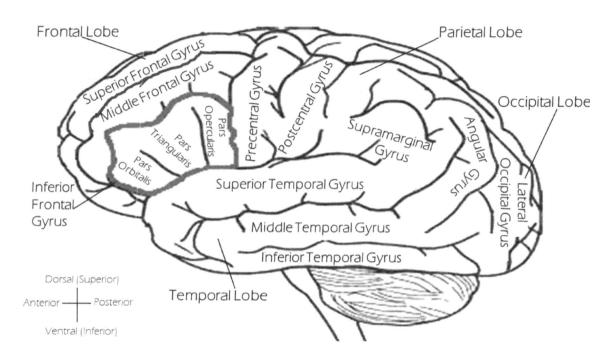

Frontal Lobe

Superior Frontal Gyrus

Middle Frontal Gyrus

Pars Opercularis

Pars Triangularis

Pars Orbitalis

Precentral Gyrus

Postcentral Gyrus

Parietal Lobe

Supramarginal Gyrus

Angular Gyrus

Occipital Lobe

Lateral Occipital Gyrus

Inferior Frontal Gyrus

Superior Temporal Gyrus

Middle Temporal Gyrus

Inferior Temporal Gyrus

Temporal Lobe

Dorsal (Superior)

Anterior — Posterior

Ventral (Inferior)

Brain cortex: frontal, parietal, temporal and occipital lobes and what they do

First, a quiz question. If you suffer a blow to the head, which part of your brain is most likely to be affected? Since much head trauma comes from events like being hit in the head by a baseball, or falling off a bike, you might guess that the front part of your brain may take the brunt of a blow, and you would be correct statistically.

But let 's take a closer look at the complex anatomy and function of the brain, remembering that medical science doesn't know nearly enough about the brain and nervous system, and that the responsibilities of various parts of the brain often overlap functionally!

To start with, the brain cortex, that cauliflower-like structure right under your skull, has four lobes, each lobe with a right and left side and each lobe with different but complementary functions. The right and left sides of our cauliflower-like brains are separated from each other by fissures but connected by a structure tucked underneath called the Corpus Callosum. The corpus callosum is a thick bundle of nerve fibers connecting and integrating the activities of the halves of the cortex, such as vision.

If you are an unfortunate baby born without your corpus callosum, and some babies are, you can have big problems. You may be developmentally delayed, have difficulty with using language and recognizing social cues like friendliness and anger, and you may even have an unusual face.

Back to the lobes of the brain. Mr. L, who was only in his early sixties, was a growing embarrassment to his family. Though his memory was good, this once reliable and devoted husband and father said and did inappropriate sexual things. He could no longer do his job, which required concentration and attention to detail. The nurses at the clinic where he went for his medical problems were now afraid to take his blood pressure, pulse and respiratory rate because his hands went where they shouldn't and his risqué vocabulary was readily understood by the medical personnel, almost all of whom were fairly fluent in Spanish.

Mr. L was a victim of frontotemporal dementia. His plight, which sometimes has genetic roots, emphasizes some of the fallout from having an illness which destroys one's frontal lobes. The frontal lobes play an important role in concentration, attention, planning, speech fluency, and sexual function. Problems in certain areas can even cause a spastic paralysis.

To illustrate further, there is the fascinating story of Phineas Gage. As a young man, this farm boy took a job as foreman on a railroad building crew way back in time when the railroads were just being constructed in the US. While trying to dynamite an obstreperous rock, his tamping rod, which was used to position the explosive underneath the rock, somehow caused ignition. The rod thereupon was driven from his left lower cheekbone through the left frontal lobe of his brain, only to exit through the top of his skull and become airborn for several more yards. Though he returned afterward to work, his fellow laborers noticed such a significant change in his personality that he seemed to them to be "no longer Gage". He had become "restless, disrespectful and unreliable". He also created a sensation in the medical community because his injury clearly showed that structural brain problems can impact personality!

The story ends rather better than it started. His brain's plasticity was demonstrated by the fact that he was not only able to support himself through work for the rest of his life, but his personality began to slowly improve too! (30) (www.britannica.com/biography/Phineas-Gage)

Frontotemporal dementia also involves the temporal lobes. These bilateral lobes are tucked in the bottom middle lobe of the cortex, and the upper surfaces of the temporal lobes on either side are next to all three other lobes. The temporal lobes therefore are under your skull roughly above your earlobes. Their function relates to hearing and to interpreting what is heard. The temporal lobes also play a part in smell, in vision, and in emotions. Disorders (lesions) in discrete parts of the temporal lobes cause different problems. For example, if you are right handed and have a lesion, or disorder, in a part of the left temporal lobe and adjacent parietal lobe, you won't be able to understand spoken speech, won't be able to read or repeat sounds or words, and may not be able to write. However you yourself may actually speak fluently! (31) (Mohr, J.P., Disorders of speech and language, pp156-162 in Harrison's Principles of Internal Medicine, Thirteenth Edition, Isselbacher, Kurt J. et al, Mcgraw-hill, Inc 1994)

The parietal lobe sits in the top middle part of the brain. Its job is to perceive and integrate signals from sensory nerves like touch, temperature, position, and special organization. It also plays a role in interpreting body language.

The occipital lobe interprets visual sensations, perception and interpretation. It sits in the back of the cortex. However, just as in other brain functions, parts and subdivisions of the other lobes participate in sight. For example, problems or injuries in the parietal, temporal or occipital areas of the brain all can affect parts of visual perception and interpretation, such as appreciating color, understanding movement and even writing. Not only that, but subdivisions of the various lobes also have different functions. Destruction of just a portion of the visual part of the occipital lobe for instance, can cause visual hallucinations. You can appreciate that with all the overlaps of function, and with the yet unknown complexities of the cortex, neurologists (physicians who deal with the nervous system) must sometimes feel like the Lewis and Clarks of medicine.

The cerebellum sits like a little mushroom under the occipital lobe of the brain. If you are great at basketball, or a ballerina, or a construction worker plying your skill on a high-rise building, thank your cerebellum. This structure is responsible for your equilibrium, coordination, balance, and muscle tone. It also coordinates your eye movements

If the above overview leaves you dissatisfied, you are not alone. The undisputable fact is that we have a lot to learn about brain function. Because of the interweaving of structure and function between brain parts and predicated upon our constantly expanding knowledge of brain function, crude definitions are in order for other structures affiliated with the brain

The thalamus, situated in a portion of brain known as the diencephalon or upper part of the brainstem, has a "gatekeeper "function in relaying information from the body's sensory nerves (neurons) to the cerebral cortex. Problems in this relay station can affect everything from speech to sensation.

The hypothalamus is a small but important brain structure lying below the thalamus and in connection with the pituitary gland. It makes neurohormones which "give orders" to the pituitary gland by way of a connecting stalk. In essence, it is a kind of bridge between the neural and endocrine systems . But wait, there's more! This walnut sized structure, found in all creatures with a backbone, maintains body homeostasis. That includes everything from temperature to being hungry!

The pituitary, which sits between the nerves of vision (optic nerves) on their journey to the occipital lobe, is below the hypothalamus and connected to it by the aforementioned stalk, which sends chemical messengers to the back part (posterior pituitary) of the pea sized pituitary. The pituitary is divided into anterior and posterior sections with different hormonal duties. If you feel lethargic, are gaining weight, are constipated, have muscle aches and generally aren't your former active self, it could be your pituitary…or your thyroid…or something completely different like your mother in law's cooking.

The anterior pituitary produces a bunch of hormones whose duty it is to provide feedback to other endocrine glands. Thyroid stimulating hormone (TSH) is secreted or produced when the thyroid gland isn't making enough thyroid hormone, luteinizing hormone (LH) helps the ovary to release an egg that when fertilized will grow into your daughter or son, and follicle stimulating hormone (FSH) tells the ovary to begin growing that egg in the first place. When the ovaries fail at menopause, FSH and LH are produced in large quantities to badger the dying ovaries back to life. Men also are involved as FSH and LH are important in sperm production. Adrenocorticotropic hormone or ACTH instructs the adrenal gland to produce cortisol in just the proper amounts. Prolactin is important for milk production in the pregnant and breast-feeding mom.

Then we have the posterior pituitary, whose production of growth hormone or GH, regulates growth and a whole lot of other things like glucose metabolism. Oxytocin, another hormone produced in the posterior pituitary, helps the uterus get back to normal after pregnancy and also opens the milk channels so babies can be fed breast milk

The basal ganglia, a group of neurons below the cortex, and deep inside the brain, specialize in learning and in fine tuning specific motor activities, and so receives and processes information from other brain areas. Steph Curry probably has extraordinary basal ganglia, but people with Parkinson's disease, not so much.

Now we travel downward to the medulla, without which you would not be alive at all. Anatomically, it sits atop the spinal cord and is responsible for all the life sustaining functions your body carries out without your even thinking about it. It regulates your breathing, your heart function, the coordination of swallowing, your blood pressure, all those autonomic or self-sustaining functions that let you keep alive. The pons, a waystation transmitting messages from the lower to upper brain, sits right above the medulla, and plays a part in rapid eye movement (REM) sleep. (30)(www.thebrainmadesimple.com) The reticular activating system is a clump of neurons regulating sleep and arousal and the transition from one state to another. This would be an important function if you were a caveman living in lion country, or a person who had to respond to an alarm clock to get to class on time.

If all this brain anatomy and function is confusing to you, it is confusing even to neuroscientists, who are still trying to work out the exact functions and locations of different parts of the brain. To make things even more complicated, the brain is a great shape shifter. Rewiring can take place over time if some neurons are damaged…or even if a person was born without certain structures! For example, some people born with defects in the corpus callosum, that bundle of fibers uniting the right and left hemispheres of the brain, can develop other connections and function well enough.

There was a young medical student who once long ago took a deep dive into a shallow pool. The inevitable happened, injuring his spinal cord so high up that he couldn't use his extremities. Luckily, he could still breathe. Being an individual of extraordinary perseverance, he did finish medical school, and went on to become a psychiatrist. But that isn't the end of the story. He turned to writing, then became a talking head on television. You may not have liked his political views, but you would have to respect the courage of Charles Krauthammer.

Or to cite another deceased individual with opposite political leanings but with the same courage, look to our 25th (?) president, Franklyn D. Roosevelt. After his spinal cord was damaged in a different way by the ravishes of polio, he couldn't use his legs. Knowing that he had to appear a tower of strength during World War II, he didn't allow his diplegia (loss of the use of his legs) to become evident. Photographs were always taken in such a way that his inability to walk wasn't apparent.

What is the spinal cord?

If the brain is your command organ, the orders it gives must get down to the muscles, glands, even the blood vessels, heart and stomach. The vehicle for most of this heavy lifting is the spinal cord. Think of it as containing the high voltage lines that get generated electricity to your toaster, washing machine, and lamps .

The spinal cord, a part of the central nervous system, situated below the brain, travels from the medulla all the way down to the level of the first to second lumbar vertebrae of your back. Place your hands on the top of your hip bone to locate the approximate level at which the spinal cord ends. Just as the brain is bathed in protective fluid within membranes and encased in the tough cranial bones, so too is the spinal cord protected by the vertebrae. The engineering of the protective housing of the spinal cord is a structural masterpiece, allowing for flexibility while optimizing protection. In the front, the vertebral bodies are separated from each other by the vertebral discs, non-bony structures which give flexibility and cushioning to the spine. The bones of the vertebral arch form the sides and posterior of the spine and provide spaces for the emergence of nerves from the spinal cord. In the middle of this structure is created a protected hole through which runs the delicate spinal cord, containing the nerves carrying instructions from the brain to the muscles, organs and other parts of the body. (31) (https://techmeanatomy.info/back/vertebral-column/)

Unfortunately, as we age, the bony encasement protecting the spinal cord can deteriorate, and impact the nervous "wiring".

Mr. X was an example. He'd been a construction worker, a big guy used to carry heavy loads, and eventually he became foreman of his crew. Then he retired, he REALLY retired. He put on weight and lost the muscularity he'd had in his younger days. His tummy paunch got paunchier. Eventually, he noticed worsening low back pain spreading into his buttocks on both sides. Sitting felt better than standing. His wife noticed that when they went to the supermarket, he always wanted to push the grocery cart, a chore he had previously avoided. Pushing the cart allowed him to lean forward, relieving some of his back pain. Mr X had lumbar spinal stenosis. Spinal stenosis can occur in other areas of the spine, and results from narrowing of either the central or lateral parts of the spinal canal. This can happen when osteophytes, or bony outcroppings, which are somewhat like icicles hanging off a frozen roof or stalactites dripping down from the ceiling of a wet cave, push on the nerve roots coming off the spinal cord. In some cases the contents of a vertebral disc will rupture or push into the spinal cord itself. When Mr X was sitting flexed or leaning forward, his lumbar spinal canal widened just a bit, relieving pain. When he was walking, and his spinal canal volume was reduced slightly, the pain returned. Eventually, because this encroachment upon the spinal canal tends to be progressive, Mr. X will need either a rolling walker with an attached seat or surgery.

On the other hand, Mrs B, in her late seventies, was definitely getting shorter. One day she had severe pain deep in her back, also worsened by standing but relieved by lying down. A prompt visit to her doctor followed by xrays revealed she had a compression fracture of one of her vertebrae. She got much better over the course of a month, aided by prompt treatment of the osteoporosis which had caused the compression fracture in the first place. Her increasingly fragile bones also put her at risk for more fractures . (Leo M. Cooney, Jr, MD, Chapter 57m Musculoskeletal Pain,

PP538-547. In Geriatric Review Syllabus, 9th ed, Annette Medina-Walpole. MD, AGSF, et al, 2016, American Geriatric Society)

The Peripheral Nervous System: and you thought the brain was complex!

Back to anatomy, briefly. The spinal nerves coming from the spinal cord generally pass through the intervertebral foramina, spaces in the spinal column where nerves from the spinal cord exit. Each spinal nerve has a ventral or motor root and a dorsal or sensory root. The anatomy gets complex and varies somewhat from the top of the spine, but the main concept is that different nerves have different functions. Efferent or motor nerves are those carrying instructions from the brain to various body structures like muscles, while afferent or sensory nerves are bringing information from the stimulation of sensory end organs like the skin back to the brain for analysis and possible action. These nerves are part of the peripheral nervous system which is composed of nerve fibers, ganglia and end organs. (32)((Gray's Anatomy, Thirtieth American Edition, ed. Carmine D. Clemente, AB, MS, PhD, Williams and Wilkins, Baltimore. Chapter 12, The Peripheral Nervous System, pp 1149-1282)

WE can't forget the cranial nerves which are attached to the base of the brain and exit the cranial cavity through openings in and about the skull. There are twelve of these, dealing with vision, smell, positional sense, balance, taste, swallowing, hearing and the movement of our complex facial muscles.

The Autonomic Nervous System: when, what, who, where, when

If we had to consciously think about breathing, digesting, and so forth, we couldn't function at all. The Ancients were aware of this fact and gave us the mythical story of Ondine's curse. Ondine was a beautiful water nymph who fell in love with a mortal man and thus assumed the burden of mortals, that of aging. Unfortunately, Philemon, her lover, didn't much like the fact that her beauty was fading, and set his eyes on other, younger females. So, in retaliation for being forsaken, Ondine placed a curse on him. He would stop breathing should he fall asleep!

There is a medical condition called Ondine's curse disease, or central hypoventilation syndrome, where individuals don't breathe normally when asleep. They "forget" to breathe. Babies born with this condition can be helped with assisted ventilation but sometimes have difficulties with other functions of the autonomic nervous system besides autonomic respiration..

So, what exactly is the autonomic nervous system?

Bodily functions that sustain life go on whether we are thinking about them or not, whether we are awake or asleep, or engaged in an activity that totally occupies our conscious awareness. We have our autonomic nervous systems to thank for relieving us from the work of getting our food to digest, or our hearts to pump faster when we are running to catch an airplane.

Our autonomic, or visceral, nervous system is a part of the peripheral nervous system with the whole complex of fibers, nerves, ganglia and plexuses that that affiliation implies. It is the vehicle through which information from the central nervous system (brain and spinal cord) is conveyed from and to our viscera…. organs, blood vessels, heart, even glands like the salivary glands. If we had to input consciously all the programming our autonomic nervous system does for us, we would simply not be able to. After all, Philemon died just because of autonomic nervous system failure in one domain, that of sleeping respiration!

The take home lesson is that we really don't know all there is to know about the complexity of our nervous systems, though many people are diligently working to unlock its function. New knowledge may help us make better decisions in everything from engineering to the social sciences. For example, the NIH has lately reported that persons with a genetic variation of the AKT-1 gene have an increased risk of developing psychosis with daily use of marijuana. This information is probably just the tip of the iceberg when it comes to individual genetic variations on the way the brain works…or doesn't!

How nerves work

Most everyone has seen pictures of nerve cells or neurons. They look a bit like deformed octopi, with a central body holding the cellular nucleus, a bunch of tentacles called dendrites extending in diverse directions, and a long major branching fiber called the axon. The grey matter of our brains is composed largely of the neuron cells themselves, whereas the white matter contains that long axon, usually "insulated" with a myelin sheath. Of course, there are a lot of supporting cells in the nervous system, that have various functions. To name a few, oligodendrocytes build and maintain the myelin sheathes which provide insulation for neurons. Astrocytes have housekeeping duties including those they do for the blood vessels in the central nervous system.

How communication takes place: the chemical messengers

Neurotransmitters are chemical messengers that bring messages or impulses across the gap or synapse between one neuron and the next. Some drugs used for maladies such as depression act to increase these chemical messengers.

Hormones are chemical messengers that travel long distance, not just across synapses. They are sent from a structure like the brain, or another organ like the adrenal gland, usually through the blood stream, to inform a receptor organ or gland to do something or refrain from doing something.

Mrs. J thought she must be going through an especially pernicious menopause, even though she was just 38 and her mother's menses didn't stop till age 53. She felt awful in the mornings. Her hair was falling out. Her muscles ached. She was constipated. Her periods were, in fact longer and heavier than usual. Her skin was dry and itchy. Her memory was failing. No hot flashes, though. In fact, she was cold all the time.

Her problem turned out to be a thyroid gland that was not being stimulated by another needed hormone called thyroid stimulating hormone, or TSH. TSH is manufactured in the brain and travels by attachment to a protein, called thyroid binding globulin, to stimulate the cells in the thyroid. These thyroid cells need to make precisely the appropriate amount of thyroid hormone to meet the needs of all the cells in the body. If these cells make too little, or too much thyroid hormone, problems will occur. This feedback between the brain and the thyroid maintains body homeostasis because every cell in the body is affected by thyroid hormone for better or worse. The heart and blood vessels are also impacted by thyroid hormone. With too little hormone, the heart beats slower and the blood pressure generally runs a bit lower. With too much, the heartrate is on average higher, and the systolic blood pressure can become quite high. Even cholesterol is affected, with levels tending to rise when people don't have enough circulating thyroid hormone.

Mrs J's story has a happy ending. With a tablet of replacement levothyroxine, she had resolution of all her symptoms and became a happy, normally menstruating, camper.

Growth, pruning and death of nerves

Scientists not long ago thought that we had our complete complement of neurons (nerves) when we were born or at least by early childhood. Like so many scientific ideas we have had, ideas are constantly being disproven or expanded on. For example, for you who love geology, before the 1950's, continental drift was just a theory. Nowadays, plate tectonics is the explanation for the fact that the Pacific plate is migrating in a Northwest direction about 2.75 inches a year. In fact, the Hawaiinan archipelago is birthing a new island that, may poke through the ocean in tens of thousands of years. It even has a name: Lo 'ihi.

But back to neurons. The good news is that neurons or parts of them probably can and do regenerate. According to the National Institute of Neurological Disorders and Stroke, this theory of regeneration has already been proven in such disparate creatures as the rat and the canary. We do know that learning can and does happen into old age. However, it is felt that the learning areas of the brain are at the synapses where neurons communicate with other neurons, and how this happens again is under active investigation. The bottom line however, is that old age is not a contraindication to acquiring new knowledge, though it certainly is more difficult to learn a new language at 80 than when your brain was most structurally receptive to learning communication skills, somewhere between when you were 2 months and a handful of years of age! Neurons also die, and for many reasons. A stroke will cause a cessation in the flow of food and water to neurons. Other events leading to cell death, like Alzheimer's are under vigorous investigation. Programmed neuronal cell death, called apoptosis, occurs during neuronal development as a way of structuring the CNS efficiently. Neural pruning is the way the brain gets rid of neural connections it no longer needs and occurs especially during childhood through adolescence. This pruning process is akin to pruning your rose bush so it will produce more new buds and branches! All these events concerning neurons are actively being investigated. Some day, knowing more about the life cycle of neurons may help all of us remain active and able to easily acquire new skills into old age. We are certainly not there yet!

Speaking of aging, what happens to the brain and nervous system as we age?

You are probably familiar with the saying, "You can't teach an old dog new tricks". You are probably also aware of news stories about octogenerians who have finally earned their bachelors' degrees after putting aside their educational aspirations for decades to raise and provide sustenance for their families. Then there are people like Maurine Kornfeld, a 97 year old woman whose world records in US Masters Championship competitions (national age group champion in the backstroke) belie the fact that she started swimming seriously around age 60. She reportedly didn't learn the art of putting her face in the water till retirement age.

Perhaps a brief look at the physiologic factors which could impact the ability to learn new material as we age would be helpful However, research hasn't advanced terribly much in this arena: moreover we cannot measure motivation, a crucial factor in learning. What is known is that skills and knowledge that are familiar are usually well preserved. Vocabulary and general knowledge actually improve a bit through the seventh decade. (32)(Salthouse, T. Consequences of age-related declines. Annu.Rev.Psychol 2012:63;201) Speed of processing information, however, decreases with aging. (33) (Cognitive Neuroscience of Aging: Linking cognitive and Cerebral Aging; Cabeza, R, Nybery, L., Park, D (Eds) Oxford University Press, New York 2004) The ability to remember things, to tap our memory for the information needed to do something like putting together a multi-ingredient meal and the speed with which we can recall information (processing speed) all slow down a bit as people age, along with a skill called "executive function" . Executive function is a planning and synthesizing skill usually requiring more "long term" thinking. An example might be planning a party, which requires deciding on the date, locating a physical space, drawing up a guest list and managing the list, providing food. You get the idea. Multi-tasking and tasks requiring attention slow down too.

Although learning is apparently slowed down by physiologic changes, some learning issues may be affected by the environment and by interest. Retirees may get out of practice because their environments may not make demands upon them. Interests may narrow. A study done by resident physicians queried persons over 65 about their use of electronic communications like e-mail, texting and Facebook, snapchat etc. Although access was a factor in learning new communication skills, so was a lack of desire to do so.

Curiously but perhaps not unexpectedly, considering all the other benefits of exercise, aerobic exercise seemed, in one study, not only to provide better availability of oxygen, which all neurons and other cells need to function, but also to increase verbal fluency, a language continuity skill. (34)(Noera, J et al, Changes in Cortical Activation Patterns in Language Areas following an Aerobic Exercise Intervention in Older Adults, in Neural Plasticity 2017, Academic Editor: Thomas Platz)

PET scans and even newer imaging methods are slowly opening windows on the function and even the chemical happenings in our brains, but such tools are still in their infancy. Though the aging process affects all our organs, including the central nervous system, it is known that new nerve cells (grey matter colloquially) continue to form throughout life, and they also continue to connect with each other, (35) (George E. Taffet, MD, Normal aging, PP56-57, in Up to Date,

Kenneth E. Schmader, Section Editor, Jane Givens, MD, Deputy Editor,, Feb 2019) So old dogs can learn new tricks, although they will have to put a larger part of their brains in to the learning effort, and it may take a bit longer than it would have during their puppyhood!

Normal and abnormal forgetting

We all normally lose nerve cells or neurons from apoptosis or programmed cell death. This pruning process begins in the womb and seems crucial for normal development. However, neurons in the cerebral cortex and the cerebellum seem to commit this form of "cell suicide" at a higher rate than cells in other parts of the brain. Older neurons also seem to engage each other less reliably due to loss of their dendrites and synapses Hence, forgetting the proper word or the name of an acquaintance is a common and embarrassing problem as we age.

Dr. T taught medical students and newly minted physicians. Knowing the medical material was not an issue. Occasionally pulling up the precise technical name or term was. Dr T knew that waiting a few minutes would permit the term to pop into memory. The embarrassment of having to talk around the topic or term until this process happened, however, was infuriating and embarrassing!

Dr. T's experience reflects the anatomic fact, witnessed during functional brain imaging, that the older brain must work harder, and involve more neurons for a given task. (36)(A Cognitive Neuroscience of Aging: Linking Cognitive and Cerebral Aging< Cabeza, R and Nyberg, L, Park, D (Eds) Oxford University Press, New York 2004)

Older folk worry about forgetting, feeling that any lapse in this area signals the onset of conditions like Alzheimer's Disease.

A patient, aged 67, was seated in an examining room, frantically scribbling away at a word-finding puzzle, and very upset at being interrupted. When asked what she was doing, she remarked testily that puzzles were her attempt to stave off dementia, thank you very much!

Although mild neurocognitive delay, a condition where there is a measurable decline in some aspect of cognitive or thinking function, can go on to develop into full blown dementia, it doesn't necessarily do so, or may take a considerable while to do so. However, as opposed to very mild or normal forgetfulness, this second stage becomes evident to others. It is not just a worry item for the older person who is sure he is headed for a nursing home because he mislaid his keys.

Brain shrinkage and its effects

Unfortunately, due to neuronal dropout, and changes in other brain tissues, our brains shrink as we age. This happens even in normal folk. In fact, the white matter, where the myelinated (protectively sheathed) axons live, loses more material that the grey cerebral cortex, where neurons hang out. The axons, those neuronal tails dangling from the neurons themselves, maintain communication between parts of the brain, and also send messages from the brain to the spinal cord to give orders to other parts of the body like the muscles. Cerebral blood flow, which supplies energy and oxygen to the brain, also decreases.

The net effect is brain shrinkage. This shrinkage can be seen quite vividly on MRI scans of the brain.

Unfortunately, brain shrinkage seems to make older people much more vulnerable to brain trauma. A fall can put far more tension on blood vessels and brain where there is a gap between brain and skull. Think of a bell clapper. It must be separated from the bell which houses it for ringing it to make a sound.

A seventy-year-old visiting her daughter's family for Christmas in another state, had climbed a few rungs up a small ladder to reach an object in a closet. She lost her footing and tripped, hitting her head on a hard wood floor. At first, she felt ok except for a headache, but things got worse, and she was found to have a subdural hematoma (bleed). This kind of a bleed apparently takes place when the delicate veins bridging between the two outermost of the three membranes covering the brain (named dura and subarachnoid) get torn, usually traumatically. This poor lady's visit extended not to New Year, but all the way to St. Patrick's Day (March 17th) Had it been her granddaughter's nice plump brain which sustained the force of this rather short-distance fall, no noticeable injury would have occurred.

Keeping the brain at maximal function as it ages.

Have you noticed how most earth-shattering discoveries are made by the young?

Albert Einstein worked on his theory of relativity between the ages od 23 and 30. Christopher Columbus, whatever you may think of him, was elderly 35 when he finally persuaded Queen Isabella to consider outfitting a voyage to Asia!

Charles Darwin, at age 29, had already thought out his theory of evolution.

The illiterate peasant girl, Joan of Arc, was only 16 when she started on the path to energize the French army to liberate France, actually leading them and bringing about a French victory at the Siege of Orleans

Marie Curie was only 31 when she presented her work on radioactivity to the Academie des Sciences, and was at the time a mother of a one year old.

Alexander the Great had created the largest empire in the ancient world by age 30.

Eli Whitney, whose invention of the cotton gin when he was 28 served to prolong the institution of slavery in the US (not his intention), also invented the concept of interchangeable machine parts, shoring up the Industrial Revolution.

DR. Charles Drew, the African American surgeon who developed ways of storing blood plasma and started the concept of blood banking early in World War II, was in his late 30's and early 40's when his contributions to blood banking saved the lives of unknown numbers of American and British military.

You get the idea!

WE are living much longer than did most people in the ancient world, the Middle Ages, even the 1900's. How can we promote brain health as aging and loss of neurons and other neurologic structures inevitably occurs? Backed up by research, however insufficient, the interventions that keep us healthy throughout life are those that keep our brains healthy into old age. These interventions include securing long-lived healthy progenitors (ancestors, especially parents), keeping on the thin side, exercising most every day, eating veggies and more plant than animal based foods, having lots of friends and enjoying their company often, and avoiding bad habits like smoking (yes even marijuana), drinking in excess, doing drugs, avoiding risky behaviors, working our brains daily, and probably, driving in cities at rush hour, although the latter is as yet unproven.

Bad things that happen to our brains and nervous systems

Strokes are generally bad. There are two major types of strokes, and a significant number of conditions, like hemiplegic migranes, that can mimic strokes.

Charlie was a notable figure in his small town, with his own business and membership in all the fraternal organizations the town offered. He had a family, a couple of grandkids, loved to fish and hunt, but one day in the summer of his seventy sixth year, his life abruptly changed. He woke up with serious weakness of his right side, unable to move or feel that half of his body, and he couldn't even talk properly to call for help.A right handed guy with a dominant left middle lobe, he had blocked perfusion of his middle cerebral artery at some point during the night. Charlie had an ischemic stroke, which meant that a major blood vessel to the brain became blocked or occluded. About eighty percent of strokes are due to such blockages, although in countries like China, more strokes are due to hemorrhage from a blood vessel. About 1 in 4 ischemic strokes are caused by blockage from debris or clots flipped off from the heart.

Neurologists can roughly determine the site and extent of blood vessel involvement and of nerve damage, from an anatomic knowledge of what blood vessels feed what parts of the brain. We now have "clot busters" "that under strictly defined conditions, can be used to reopen circulation and resupply oxygen and glucose before affected nerves become irreparably damaged. This is why when any sudden nerve malfunction becomes evident, 911 or similar emergency alerting systems should be called for immediate care. This care must take place in a hospital set up to do so, because a CT scan of the brain must be done prior to administration of the "clot busting "medication. If the stroke is hemorrhagic on the head CT scan, this mode of treatment is contraindicated.

Unfortunately, Charlie had his stroke over a half century ago, before CT scans, "clot buster" infusions and even stroke rehabilitation existed. He had never gotten his high blood pressure, a risk factor for heart attacks and strokes, treated. His high cholesterol wasn't addressed......he ate the high fat, meat, gravy and potatoes diet prevalent in his part of the country. His only exercise was a couple of hunting and fishing trips a year. Charlie lingered for a few weeks in the town's old-fashioned hospital whose main business was delivering the town's babies, and then he died.

Charlie was the grandfather I never really got to know. WE have come a long way in the last fifty something years, but early recognition and intervention, and even more appropriately, avoidance of the conditions leading to strokes is now the main strategy for saving and rehabilitating lives.

What about dementia, one of the most feared occurrences in old age? There are several types of dementia, and often more than one type is wrecking damage on the brain.

The woman had been very smart. She'd matriculated from an outstanding university, had maintained her interest in current events and her hobbies while raising her family, and had warm, cheerful social skills. The family had recognized that she was forgetting things, failing to balance her check book, becoming more unable to care for herself. A daughter took her in, made sure her physical needs were attended to, and brought her for a geriatric evaluation. As it turned out, the patient and the examiner had been to the same university. When the examiner asked her something about her studies, the campus, even the mascot, she would affably make a noncommittal remark, like "oh, yes", "that was fun" or "those were the days" Demented though she was, the woman was able to hoodwink the examiner for quite a while. Imagine the examiner's chagrin when the patient scored horribly on scientifically validated tests for dementia!

Differentiating the types and stages of dementia can be helpful genetically, and can help with care, but ultimately we know little about causation and even less about treatment. Many people, as noted above, may also have more than one reason for their dementia.

Persons who go on to develop Alzheimer's may begin with an entity called mild cognitive impairment. These persons will know something just isn't as it was, may notice a decline in their ability to attend to several issues at once, to learn new material, to pay bills. Their formally sharp memories may become blunted, making word-finding a chore. However, these subjective deficits don't really cause much of a problem in independent living. Although about half of persons with memory loss may progress to greater deficits, the other half don't seem to progress much over several years.

Alzheimer's disease itself is usually slowly progressive over about a decade, and many afflicted folk have a genetic marker, APOE4. Memory loss becomes worse and worse, victims become easily disoriented, forget how to do simple chores like making toast, can't remember the past, don't recognize loved ones or misidentify them, and then finally becomes nonverbal and non-ambulatory.

One of the saddest examples of decline happened to a couple who fell in love at a time when African American/Caucasian marriages were socially taboo. Nonetheless, the couple stayed strongly devoted to each other over many decades. Then the husband developed Alzheimer's, deteriorated, and eventually became confined to a wheelchair, so bad was his apraxia (loss of motor control). One day, the aged wife rolled him into a clinic, tears rolling down her cheeks, demanding that he be restored medically to his former self. She was told that the drooling, nonverbal person she so lovingly cared for over so many decades was close to death, and that no medical interventions could restore him to the vibrant strong man he had once been, and actually still was in her eyes!

Frontotemporal dementia usually strikes at a younger age than does Alzheimer's.

Mr. S was an embarrassment to his family. He just couldn't be brought anywhere, was hypersexual and disinhibited and scared all the nurses. And he was only in his early sixties! Although his memory wasn't so bad, he had trouble with the English he had formerly mastered. Now the same subtle language problems were affecting his native Spanish. Mr. S. had frontotemporal dementia, in which social propriety is lost even before memory issues become a problem. Imaging of the brain may show loss in the frontal and temporal lobes, and decline is speedier than in Alzheimer's.

Dementia with Lewy bodies can be subtle initially.Mrs. S was a gentle widow, the kind of person who brightens others' days by reveling in the joys of life. She was being examined for possible Parkinson's Disease when she innocently mentioned the little night-time visitors to her apartment. These children were silent, never took any food or messed up the furniture, and in fact she rather enjoyed their presence but had no idea how they got into her home when the door was usually locked.

Dementia with Lewy bodies involves a triad of detailed visual hallucinations, early Parkinsonian symptoms like the cogwheeling (jerkiness with flexion) of one leg that Mrs S had, and fluctuations in severity. If Parkinson's has been present for more than a year prior to the appearance of the above symptoms, then the diagnosis is Parkinson disease dementia. (37) (Alexander W. Threlfall, MD, MA and Cynthia Barton, RN, MSN, Chapter 36: Dementia, in Geriatric Review Syllabus,, 9th ed, 2016, American Geriatric Society)

Vascular dementia often occurs together with Alzheimer's. Mrs T was a mess. She had to be helped to walk, couldn't express her needs, was disheveled and had a cellulitis (bacterial skin infection) in her thigh that needed attention. She wasn't homeless, in fact she had a wealthy but disinterested family. Prior caregivers hadn't worked out, so they hired a young girl from "the other side of town". This young lady was one of the most talented caregivers ever. She was kind but strict, and rehabilitated Mrs. T with a loving discipline that usually only mothers of small children possess. Observing every detail of Mrs. T's life, she soon added a daily schedule under which Mrs. T flourished. The cellulitis healed quickly, a healthy diet was enforced, and to everyone's amazement, Mrs. T learned to ambulate and to express her needs again. Moreover, she was clean, manicured and happy.

Mrs T had multi-infarct dementia, and her downward course was like walking a staircase. With every mini stroke she regressed, got a bit better and then had another. Her new caregiver did for her the things one needs to do to prevent further strokes. Her blood pressure medications were given on schedule, her diet was vastly improved, an exercise program allowed for a slow return of her motor (muscle and bone) function, she was kept clean and infection free. Moreover, she had a caretaker who really cared that she was getting better and kept her interested in life by doing little things like taking her on walks. (many times, an unrecognized depression is a part of a stroke, interfering with the motivation to recover)

As is apparent, types of dementia often overlap or occur together, and symptoms of early dementia overlap with phenomena of normal aging. Some medications like so called cholinesterase inhibitors may temporarily suppress the advancement of symptoms, and treatment of those conditions which mimic dementia, like severe hypothyroidism, or one form of fluid on the brain (hydrocephalus) can help some folk, but by and large we face a crisis as more people get older and are at risk. Treatments which may help include things like creating a familiar environment for the sufferer, having repetative reassuring daily routines, and treating the pain, depression and discomfort that often the patient her or himself can't articulate. Always we need to remember that the whole family suffers too!

Delerium is another bad actor, often occurring when an older person is taken out of his regular routine and is faced with illness or surgery. This condition is seen quite commonly in sick, hospitalized patients. Mr T had always liked hunting. He had a small collection of guns accumulated over a lifetime, and as a responsible father and good citizen, kept them locked up.

When he retired, and especially after his wife died, Mr. D began "losing it". His daughter was very concerned about incipient dementia, because Mr T had become a bit paranoid and forgetful. Things reached a crisis level when Mr. T had to be hospitalized for an unrelated problem. Nurses noted that at times he was alert and lucid, and at other times quite confused. He mentioned his guns. His daughter said that this behavior was new, but she also reiterated her concern about creeping dementia and paranoia. Considering a diagnosis of delirium superimposed on a mild dementia, his doctor and nurse began to look for factors which may have triggered his behavior. His medications were reviewed. Some medications as seemingly innocuous as over-the-counter formulas for allergies (antihistamines like Benadryl) or stomach problems, (H2 blockers like ranitidine) can cause problems when a slightly demented person is placed in an unfamiliar, frightening place like a hospital. Mr. T was checked for hidden infections in the bladder, for constipation, for breathing issues, for fragmented sleep, for unrecognized pain. His nurse made sure that his dentures, eyeglasses and hearing aide were all available and in working shape. Noise, confusing schedules and light were kept to a minimum. Precautions were taken to prevent falls, and physical therapy was called upon to get him more active. Mr T responded to these ministrations fairly well and was ready to go home when his daughter remembered the guns. These were taken from the home and stored and Mr T's car keys were also secured.

The term "delirious" is used rather glibly, but it is a real entity, and we don't really understand all its roots or how to cure it. DSM-5, the psychiatrists" handbook, describes it as "a disorder of attention and awareness that develops acutely and tends to fluctuate". It tends to be a big problem especially for older hospitalized folk and may unmask an unsuspected early dementia. Many people who had experienced delirium while hospitalized still are affected many months later. Should the symptoms last more than six months, full recovery isn't too likely. Many hospitals have taken action to diminish the risk of delirium, by making sure a patient has access to his glasses and hearing aides, by trying to prevent falls (but not with physical restraints) by minimizing sleep disruption and being careful about medications which could cause delirium, and in a host of other ways. Even bringing familiar things from home can help!

Parkinsonian disease got a good deal of attention when Michael J. Fox, actor in thew 1985 movie "Back to the Future", became affected. The actor who had played a legendary character then became an advocate for affected persons. Other notable persons with Parkinsonism have included Muhammed Ali and several other sports figures, even an astronaut!

There are many ways the complexities of the aging neurologic system can affect people. Parkinsonian symptoms are familiar to most people, and can occur at a younger age, but are more common in the elderly. It is one of the many movement disorders which referentially affect older people.

Mr Z had longstanding Parkinson's disease. He had had all its complications: a resting tremor, very slow movements (bradykinesia) muscle rigidity and problems with ambulation including retropulsion, or a risk of moving and falling backward. His wife could hear him shuffling down the hall with his Parkinsonian gait. Medications helped quite a bit…for a while. (Carbidopa-levodopa and others) Now however, when his medication effect ran out, he would just "freeze". Also, he was beginning to show some signs of early dementia.

Many neurologic conditions can mimic Parkinson's disease, and a thorough neurologic exam is mandatory to make the correct diagnosis. In general, the four diagnostic features include slow movements, a resting tremor, rigidity of muscles, and poor postural reflexes, meaning the patient has difficulty keeping his balance. Early on, afflicted persons may have "cogwheeling" which is jerky movement when one or more extremities is passively flexed, and their writing may get much smaller than before (micrographia) Parkinson's disease can rob the victim of the normal spontaneous facial movements so necessary for social communication. Fortunately, medications can be very helpful for a long time, making an almost normal life possible. However, the neurodegeneration in the end is progressive.

Tumors and cancer

Cancer isn't one disease. It has many roots: genetic, environmental and lifestyle. The prevalence of most cancers increases as we age. Most cells in our bodies respect boundaries. Cancer cells do not: they travel or metastasize. Our body has an inborn system to attack these wandering misfits. Our immune system contains specialized cells, chemicals and proteins whose mission it is to destroy cancer cells and other invaders before they multiply and cause damage. Unfortunately, our immune system also undergoes an aging process, making most cancers more of a possibility as we grow older. Increasingly however, cancer treatments are directed at using medications allied or interacting with our own immune systems to fight some types of cancer. Other contributors, it is thought, to cancer in older folk may include more years of exposure to both natural radiation, which can damage the inner workings of cells, and teratogens, substances which promote cancer cells' growth,

Tumors are not necessarily cancerous. They are just masses and may be benign. Nonetheless, they often get in the way.

That was Mr. F's problem. He had an enlarging squishy bump on his head. It was getting in the way of combing what little hair he had left. He'd first noticed it years ago when his hair was plentiful and brown. It was a minor inconvenience, but he finally decided to get it "taken care of". Mr F's 'tumor" was a large sebaceous cyst. After total removal, Mr. F was finally able to comb his hair normally. Unfortunately, there was no improvement in hair growth. Tumors like lipomas (fat tumors) and cysts can pop up almost anywhere, but the cells comprising the tumor or cyst do not metastasize, or infiltrate into other body structures. They are not "malignant".

Several different types of cancers have their start in the brain or other parts of the nervous system. Other cancers seed the nervous system (metastasize) even though they come from other structures or parts of the body. Yet another method of attack on the central nervous system is through the production by cancer cells of chemicals or hormones which travel to the central nervous system and cause problems. And some rare cancers are very vascular (have lots of blood vessels), can get to the brain, and cause potentially fatal hemorrhage there.

It is quite apparent that nervous system cancers are quite pleomorphic and cannot be neatly characterized. We also are in the early stages of understanding the mechanisms by which cancer cells operate and are in fact realizing that each individual type of cancer will ultimately have to be fought at a molecular level.

Mrs B possessed a gene which was strongly associated with the presence of both ovarian and breast cancers. She developed cancer of the breast close to the time of menopause. Surgery was successful and she had time to raise her girls to adulthood and play with her granddaughters. Then something happened. She became confused, had trouble at work, and was finally discovered to have metastases or growths of her breast cancer in her brain and spinal cord. Immediate radiation of the spinal cord was done to prevent paralysis due to metastatic tumor growth. Things did not go well after that, and Mrs B died with her daughters at her side when she was in her early seventies. Her daughters had advanced warning and pursued genetic studies so they could take precautions against a repeat of their beloved mother's disease progression.

For some cancers we have genetic studies that will allow doctors to assess risk to family members or start screening for certain cancers early in life, so it is important for everyone to know their family histories, and act if they have known risk factors .

Encephalitis, meningitis, aneurisms, and "brain bleeds" in general are a smorgasbord of other maladies affecting the nervous system but can happen any time in the life cycle. For these conditions, antibiotics and surgery may be the answer.

Surgery on the brain was performed over 7,000 years ago, and most likely in many cases for the same reasons we do similar surgery today. The operation, called trepanation, involved drilling or scraping a hole in the head. Some of the people who had undergone this crude surgery went on to heal and to live years longer. Nothing is new under the sun!

Trauma was probably a not unexpected happening in a prehistoric person's life, and brain bleeds would have been the consequence in many cases.

Let's take a look at the coverings of the brain. From outside to inside over the brain and spinal cord, there are three membranes: the dura, arachnoid and pia maters The spinal fluid circulates between the arachnoid and the pia membranes, cushioning the brain itself from trauma. The dural veinous sinuses are veins that drain from the brain into the internal jugular vein and these veins are located between the dural layers themselves. The subarachnoid space, between the arachnoid and pia membranes, is rich in arterial blood vessels. Subarachnoid bleeds can often occur because of aneurisms or arteriovenous malformations. About 5% of the population is thought to have aneurisms, which are protrusions of weak spots in a blood vessel's wall, making rupture a possibility. Aneurisms are abnormal outward bulging in a blood vessel where its wall is weakened. Arteriovenous malformations are connections between veins and arteries, bypassing the small capillaries and these also can be prone to rupture.

Subdural hematomas are relatively common in old age. They can often become chronic and cause headache, mild cognitive problems, and sometimes specific neurologic signs, seizures, or communicating hydrocephalus which is associated with dementia. You could see why an astute caveman, recognizing the problem of a severe headache or even a traumatic neurologic abnormality, would want to perform a surgery like trepanation to get rid of the evil spirits of fluid pressure and blood and even have quite successful results!

Subarachnoid hemorrhages are usually more brutal, with a high mortality than are subdurals. Aneurisms may also increase in size over time. Sudden bleeding from rupture is said to be felt as "the worse headache of my life". . Although surgery may be needed, it is probable that the complex operations done now were beyond the sophistication of our bronze age medicine men.

One sexagenarian recalls how her funny beloved husband complained of a very severe headache, and before he could be transported to a hospital had succumbed to his massive subarachnoid bleed. She wistfully remembers how they would walk on the beach looking for shooting stars, but now such phenomenon just reminds her of her sudden terrible loss.

Encephalitis and meningitis are infections of the brain or of the above meninges respectfully. Though they are more common in babies and young children, there is another peak in seniors, again as the immune system ages and fails in its duty of attacking bacteria, viruses and fungi before they multiply and cause clinical disease.

But perhaps strokes, which can affect any area of the brain or spinal cord depending upon the blood vessel which becomes blocked or hemorrhages, are the most feared types of brain insult in all folk, especially in seniors. Today we have all sorts of tests for visualization of the brain and spinal cord, like MRI's PET scans and good old-fashioned CT's but specialists who can do an expert neurologic exam are still indispensable for an accurate diagnosis and appropriate intervention. In a stroke, when blood supply is suddenly cut off, the cells of the brain die quickly in major insult. An area around the "point of maximal impact" called the penumbra, can return to function, given proper care. Nowadays, advanced cardiac life support classes teach not only about heart emergencies but also about stroke emergencies. There are interventions, ranging from the use of "clot buster" medications like recombinant tissue -plasminogen activator (rt-PA) to endovascular thrombectomy (going through a blood vessel to get at the clot) which can save a lot of brain tissue right away. But before rescue therapy can be used, a CT must be done quickly to determine if the stroke was a hemorrhagic one, in which case clot busters would further extend the hemorrhagic or a thrombotic stroke. Time and other critical factors enter into decisions about therapy. Some hospitals are designated especially for immediate stroke evaluation and treatment. A neurologist evaluates quickly if the patient has had a probable stroke, how long ago, and what treatment is needed. And then an emergency CT of the brain is done to be sure the person hasn't had a bleeding stroke. Follow up is very important with physical therapy occupational therapy, nutrition, speech therapy when needed, and a host of other interventions to return patients to the best possible pre-stroke condition.

Attention to the psychologic needs of both patient and family is also very important. Many patients are clinically depressed after a stroke, and recognizing and treating depression plays a powerful role in return to function! Then there are the needs of the family to consider.

Mrs W was a 64-year-old African American woman who had singlehandedly raised her family, working at menial jobs and always being there for her kids. Her stroke was a bad one, involving paralysis and the inability to speak properly. While she was in the hospital, her daughter would come and clean up her stools and urine, bathe her, talk to her. The attending physician on the ward told the daughter in no uncertain terms that such care was the purvey of the nursing staff: do not interfere! Within the week, he was followed by another attending, and this attending was queried too about the daughter's interventions. The daughter tearfully explained that she didn't mind cleaning up after her mother. In fact, she wanted to do it! Her mother had sacrificed her life for her kids, and was very much loved. The daughter felt that she must give back for mom's many years of sacrifice. Caring for her allowed the daughter to express her love in a very concrete way. The daughter was happily allowed to resume care!

Depression and pseudo-depression is also not uncommon in the elderly.

Mrs X had six children. She was rather narcissistic, even at age 69, had a "boyfriend" in the senior living facility she called home, and seemed not to have any understanding of other people's needs She must have possessed this personality for a long time, because of all her children, not one of them wanted to take care of her. However, they mutually did recognize their responsibility for her welfare. Their solution? Round robin-ing Grandma. She would visit each child's family for 6 weeks, then travel on to the home of the next in line. This arrangement seemed to work…. moderately well. Mental illness and personality quirks do not necessarily resolve with advancing years and may in some cases be responsible for elder neglect. However, the mental state most likely to have an unfortunate outcome is depression.

People who have been happy and cheerful may maintain that attitude through life. That was the case with Mrs O. A giving person who always saw the best in everyone, she cared for her beloved husband as he died of cancer. She'd smile at that most menial of chores, changing diapers when his cancer had progressed to the point of incontinence, saying "I did it for our babies, I can certainly do it for him". When he died, she firmly resolved to keep herself busy and involved in life. Neighbors who could no longer drive were transported to their doctors' appointments by her. She even did wash for another ill neighbor. Occasional dinners with old friends from her former employment were a treat. All through this, her husband was always in her "thoughts and prayers". Though she was not depressed, if you asked her, she would probably tell you she longed for the time she would be with him again. Were these suicidal thoughts? Most assuredly not.

On the other hand, severe depression and suicide are real issues for many older people, and especially, white men. One elderly Caucasian man had struggled with depression and had been open to every treatment pro-offered. None had alleviated his suffering. His last recourse was electroconvulsive therapy.

Depression can also be part of organic illness, so that severe depression, not just the sadness that afflicted a woman from Mexico who didn't have the money for an air flight to visit her children, must be addressed as a part of treatment. (She did get to make the trip!) Since psychiatric disease is often a taboo topic for elderly persons, a high index of suspicion is advisable.

This most complex of all body structures, the human nervous system, has certainly eluded our efforts to understand its mysteries. Maybe we never will understand its workings completely. But there is so much more to learn, and a great many people attempting to do so.

WE await the future!

CHAPTER 10

Hormones and aging

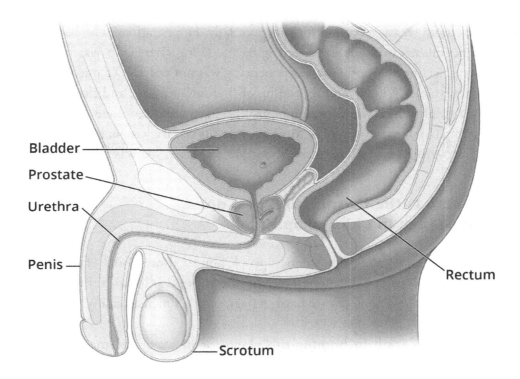

First, a definition. Hormones are chemical messengers, which usually travel through the blood stream and target organs or cells to produce an effect from these targeted structures. For example, the brain hormone, TSH, or thyroid releasing hormone, does what its name says. It tells the thyroid gland to make and release thyroid hormone. Even plants have hormones which can travel in sap and influence how a particular plant adapts to its environment. New hormones have been identified in the recent past, and this happenstance will almost certainly continue. Hormones are generally made in the endocrine glands, such as the adrenals, the ovaries and testes, and the hypothalamus, but perhaps this is too oversimplified a view. For example, vitamin D is considered not just a vitamin but also a hormone. It also has hormonal like functions. However, vitamin D production involves a multitude of organs, including the skin, and the liver and kidneys.

The thyroid and how it functions through life

Senora Y was about 60. She had been born on a ranchero in Mexico, never really learned how to read or write, worked the soil and had a dozen or so kids, some of whom had died in infancy and a couple of whom had made it to the US. One of the daughters had indeed made a life for herself and her family in California, become a citizen, married and had three children. Mrs Y was now a widow, in poor health and visiting her daughter, who was alarmed at how sedentary the vigorous mother of her youth had become. A trip to the local health center was warranted.

Mrs Y was found to have crackly breath sounds, called rales, in her lower lungs. Her legs were swollen, her heart rate was abnormal, her ability to think and recall events also reduced. She was uncomfortably constipated, had a mass in her neck, her skin was dry, her hair falling out. Walking across the exam room was a marathon for this poor lady. Her daughter, who had assumed that the changes in her mother were attributable to aging and living a harsh life, was surprised to learn that the shocking decline her mother was experiencing was not only NOT due to aging, but was in fact mostly reversable. With a careful titration of thyroid hormone, and close attention to the congestive heart failure which was the result of insufficient thyroid hormone to allow her heart to contract and pump blood effectively, Mrs Y in a few months was back to making menudo, her skin and hair were recovering and perhaps most important to Mrs Y, she was no longer constipated!

What and where is the thyroid, and how does its function change in older people?

When the conversation turns to hormones, people almost always think of the thyroid first. If one is too fat or perhaps can't gain enough weight, the fault must lie with this maligned gland. If the blood pressure is low, or stools are hard to pass, or one's menstrual cycle is all messed up, blame the thyroid.

There is a grain of truth in blaming this gland for many of the maladies which affect humankind. This gland straddles the trachea and esophagus in the front of the neck and receives its marching orders from thyroid stimulating hormone, manufactured in the hypothalamus of the brain. Sometimes the thyroid grows big and produces a bump in the front of the neck known colloquially as a goiter. Just about all the cells in the body interact with thyroid hormone. If hormone production is too high, younger folk can have blood pressure changes, a tremor, maybe diarrhea, sparse menses, weight loss, weakness in the muscles of their upper arms and thighs. Sometimes the symptoms of an overactive thyroid look like those of a panic attack.

This happened to Ms. K, a sales representative who was feeling so bad that she went to a local ER and was told she was having an anxiety attack. Not really believing this diagnosis, she followed up with a visit with her own physician, who had known her a while. Investigation revealed that the thyroid was producing too much hormone, and Ms. K was treated appropriately with medication to calm down her racing heart and to normalize hormone production.

Although the symptoms of excess thyroid hormone are relatively clear-cut in younger patients, a strange phenomenon frequently occurs in older persons. It is called apathetic thyrotoxicosis.

Although thyroid hormone levels are very high, older folk may not be hyperkinetic. Instead, they may seem depressed, withdrawn, lacking energy and may have a poor appetite, weight loss, constipation, and muscle weakness. These complaints are sometimes attributed to anorexia or depression. Heart problems often take the form of atrial fibrillation, a significant disturbance in heart rhythm that can lead to other problems like stroke. In fact, if an older person presents with atrial fibrillation, or has a phone that captures this abnormal heart rhythm, the first thing medical personnel test, after getting a corroborating electrocardiogram, is thyroid function.

Mr A was such a patient. He came in for a routine exam and his heart rate was not regular. An EKG was done, demonstrating the atrial fibrillation. Thyroid hormones were investigated. Mr. A was seen promptly by a cardiologist, who put him on one medication to regulate his rapid heart rhythm and another to prevent clots in the heart which could travel to the brain, causing a stroke. He came back saying he couldn't figure out why he had felt so tired for the past few months. Now with proper treatment he felt that his energy was back.

Sometimes the thyroid just doesn't produce enough hormone, no matter how hard the hypothalamus signals it to do so by upping the levels of TSH (thyroid stimulating hormone) being produced. Such was the case with Senora Y. Then, synthetic or animal derived thyroid hormone must be substituted.

Hypothyroidism in older individuals can sometimes be a tricky diagnosis to make. The term applies to an insufficiency of thyroid hormone to meet the needs of the body's cells. Sometimes this insufficiency is due to the brain's failure to make enough TSH (thyroid stimulating hormone) to stimulate the thyroid gland to make more thyroid hormone. This activity where one hormone promotes the production of another hormone is called a feedback loop and is seen with other hormones too. The brain once again is orchestrating homeostasis or equilibrium between the needs of the body and the timely production of quantities of hormone to exactly meet those needs. Sometimes the brain is doing its job and the thyroid or other end (producing) organ is not. Either way, the hormonal needs of the body's cells are not being met. Unfortunately, in the elderly patient, the symptoms of low thyroid production can overlap with those of depression, heart disease, Alzheimer's and a host of other maladies of aging.

A lovely but uneducated lady, Mrs T, was in her mid sixties when her routine tests done upon her visiting a new physician, showed a very high level of free calcium in her blood. Because calcium is important for muscle contraction, for bone construction, in fact for just about every aspect of cellular function, Mrs T's doctor did an extensive search for the cause of this elevated calcium level. Special bone xrays, called DEXA scans, showed that Mrs T was losing calcium from her bones. The analogy would be a house losing bricks. Mrs T was in danger of fracturing one or more of the bones in her now weakened skeleton. Of course there are many reasons for this condition, known as osteoporosis. Multiple hormones like estrogen, thyroid hormone, parathyroid hormone, vitamin D and even lifestyle factors such as smoking all influencing bone degradation. Further testing led to the finding that one or more of the four parathyroid glands sitting atop her thyroid (but having nothing to do at all with thyroid function) might be pouring out too much parathyroid hormone and leaching her bones of their calcium content. The rogue gland or glands was pouring out far too much hormone and upsetting the delicate balance of the many factors needed for bone stability. Surgery on rogue parathyroid glands solved the problem, although further medical care was needed, and Mrs T did well. Although she never quite got the gist of what was actually going on in her body, in spite of repeated explanations, she was happy with the results!

Parathyroid hormone (PTH), as noted above, is one of the many hormones and other factors which interact to assure healthy bone, muscle, and even calcium metabolism, and whose function involves organs as disparate as the gut and kidneys. Too much or too little PTH can have a devastating impact on seniors.

Another organ with feedback to the pituitary, and which is seldom given much notice, is the adrenal gland or glands, for there is one atop each kidney. The adrenal gland produces a plethora of hormones, including metanephrines, aldosterone and testosterone, but perhaps the hormone with which people are most familiar is cortisol. Following signaling from the brain (hypothalamus, pituitary) the adrenal pours out cortisol in response to stress, infection

Take Mrs G for example, she was only in her forties, but over several months, she became more and more lethargic, taking to her bed and claiming lack of energy to the point where her husband had to take over household responsibilities and the care of her teenage kids. Not only was she nauseous and anorexic, but her skin was gradually assuming a bronze tint, as though she had been sunbathing a lot. She had Addison's disease, a condition where the adrenal glands are not making enough cortisol hormone to meet daily needs. Fortunately, she was treated and regained her former energy. However, an older person may present with very nonspecific symptoms, which could easily be attributed to their advancing years, including loss of appetite, weakness, low blood pressure or maybe just failing to care for themselves properly. On the other hand, older folk paced on steroid treatment (prednisone etc) may have signs of too much cortisol, since a variety of these drugs do the same thing natural cortisol does in the body. Another cause of too much cortisol is the presence of an adenoma in the adrenal, overproducing hormone and not listening to the clues to limit production being sent by the brain. Excess cortisol really increases the risk of osteoporosis and subsequent bone fracture.

Now we get to the more problematic hormones, those secreted by the testes and ovaries.

Mr. B had come in for a physical exam. History was reviewed and revealed only an elevated blood pressure for which he was on an antihypertensive (blood pressure lowering) drug which worked well for him. After a precursory physical exam, Mr B hemmed and hawed and revealed the real reason for his visit. His wife had sent him. They had had a fulfilling sexual relationship for forty years, producing 3 children. But things had gone from bad to worse over the past year or two. Initially, erections were weak and required stimulation. Now they were nonexistent. Mr B was frustrated, embarrassed, felt he wasn't the man he used to be. Mrs B was frustrated.

Decreasing testosterone levels are common with the aging process. Depending upon the cause, be it because the brain isn't doing its job of sending hormones to stimulate production, or non response from the testes themselves, or clogged blood vessels weakening erections, or even chronic disease, ed is a common problem. However, there are solutions, depending upon the source of the problem. It is important to realize that testosterone is also a factor in bone health, so low testosterone puts men at risk of developing osteoporosis.

Estrogen and progesterone share the same feedback process with the brain, which puts out FSH and LH, hormones which spur the ovaries and regulate the production of eggs in the ovaries.

Around menopause, the ovaries lose the follicles which produce eggs, and stop listening to the brain as it sends out signals to produce estrogen, and in the second half of the female cycle, progesterone. These two hormones are responsible for the sequential maturation and release of eggs from ovarian follicles and also for the preparation of the lining of the uterus to accept the fertilized egg to grow properly into a mature baby. But that is not the only task of ovarian hormones. They also assist bone growth, influence the proper deposition of fat, promote breast maturation and do so much more! (38) (David A. Gruenewald, MD; Anne M. Kenny, MD and Alvin M. Matsumoto, MD. Chapter 63, Endocrinology, Geriatrics Review Syllabus, 9th ed. Annette Medina-Walople, MD, AGSF, James T. Pacala, MD, MS, AGSF, and Jane E. Potter, MD, AGSF, Editors-in-Chief, 2016)

Before menopause, which is the complete cessation, for at least 12 months, of the menses that mark fertility, women often have a sputtering of hormone production called the perimenopause. For most women menopause occurs statistically around age 51. AS almost everyone is aware, menopause, or the absence of meaningful levels of estrogen and progesterone, results in everything from hot flashes and poor sleep to skin changes and even weight gain. This is the time when loss of bone tissue begins in earnest.

By the time most women are 65 or older, they have accommodated to the changes, but still have to be aware of their increasingly fragile, bones, which may cause an increased risk of fractures.

WE are constantly discovering "new" hormones, which of course have been there all along. Take for example, the hormone Ghrelin. This hormone sends signals to the brain from the stomach to make you hungry! The intestines apparently will be a source of yet undiscovered hormones. We certainly have not even scratched the surface of how the gastrointestinal tract communicates with the central nervous system, how it affects sugar metabolism and many other functions. Some scientists even refer to the gastrointestinal tract t as a "second brain." More to come, which may unlock the secret to healthy weight control.

Sometimes malignant tumors can also produce incomplete hormones, which can confuse things and even cause biologic effects. Lung tumors are notorious for this.

Also, the rate at which hormones dissipate varies from person to person. Occasional women have had pregnancies well beyond the normal age for menopause, men have fathered children in old age. The oldest woman to conceive and give birth naturally, without the assistance of such technologies as IVF, was Dawn Brooke, an Englishwoman who was 59.

There was a lady on the West Coast who in her youth had a large number of children. She had come from a country where women ordinarily married in their teens At age 50 to her surprise, she gave birth to a beautiful baby girl. She had long since forgotten the details of raising a baby. Thankfully, several grown daughters with children of their own lived nearby. They apparently took turns helping their mother raise this latecoming sister!

Baring Abraham and Sara, whose ages we do not accurately know, the oldest father recorded in the Guinness Book of World Records was Les Colley whose ninth son, Oswald, was born in 1992. It is not known if genetic studies were done to document his paternity. However, older fathers have been more recently reported from other countries. As in all matters open to question, genetic verification is not stated. However, since male potency declines at a somewhat slower state than female, and since all reported elderly dads had much younger wives, the phenomenon of an older dad is a bit more believable and illustrates the disparity of hormone production in different individuals.

Be prepared for an explosion in the next few years, centered around hormones. These may be the "holy grail" of obesity research, helping us all, even those genetically programmed to gain five pounds from a single bite of food, to stay slim and fit, even in our advanced years!

CHAPTER 11

The immune System: your body's warriors

Mr. B surprised everyone. He had led a spectacular life, been a hero of sorts in World War II, raised a devoted and intelligent family, started a successful business, volunteered in several charitable organizations and had done the "dirty work" involved, not just the fun work of sitting on committees or going to fundraisers. In short, he was a man best described by that descriptive Yiddish word "Mensch".

But now he lay barely responsive in an ICU bed, fighting a terrible infection. Our medical team didn't want to give up on Mr. B. We sensed that he was the kind of guy whose whole life had shown that he wasn't the type, even in his nineties, to call it quits. So, we ignored subtle comments about hospice, as did his family. Two or three family members would arrive at the crack of dawn, to be replaced by others as the day wore on. The family had also called in spiritual reinforcements and enrolled his whole congregation in pestering the Almighty for a healthy outcome.

The Almighty must have been listening, because on the day I rotated off the ICU service, he was siting in a chair thanking the doctors-in-training, interns and residents alike, and the nurses for all they had done. His immune system had come through for him. All the antibiotics in the world would not have saved Mr. B were it not for the immune system, an incredible array of unique cells, protein messengers and other substances that prevents a small cut from ushering bacteria into the bloodstream, that fights the flu, and that even destroys funguses.

In the time of Covid19, the aging of the immune system has been brought into sharp focus for all of us. The mandated return of elderly persons, after hospitalization, to their former nursing homes has resulted in an enormous uptick in nursing home deaths. Most nursing home patients are old and frail, with the comorbidities that happen over time, and their immune systems have little reserve to fight a new virus. Science is showing us now, that recovering victims of Covid19 can excrete the virus for a week or more even when they are on the mend. Plenty of time to infect the co-inhabitants of their nursing homes, especially since viral spread seems to be abetted by incontinence.

The young and middle aged, in most cases, as the USC study is showing, can fight off this virus quickly compared with their seniors. They may not even have any signs of illness!

SO it is intuitive that the immune system, just like all our other organs, is less efficient as we age.. Anyone who has worked in an emergency room or taken care of very ill patients in a hospital quickly develops a sixth sense about which patients are more likely to survive a catastrophic illness. Besides the seriousness s of the illness, or injury, the next most important factor in survival seems to be age.

We hear a lot about "healthy hearts" and bowel function, and even erectile dysfunction, but the immune system is a black hole for most people, including scientists. Yet if not for our immune systems, we would all have died in infancy.

The immune system is our body's military, its defense system against the enemies that intrude on our physical space daily. These enemies include bacteria, viruses, prions, cancer cells that we generate within ourselves or with the help of invading viruses, worms, yeast, amoebae, and other malefactors. (39)(Peter J. Delves, PhD, University College, London, Overview of the Immune System-immunology:Allergic disorders, Merck Manual Professional Version)

However, our knowledge of the construction and function of our immune system is a process in evolution.

Perhaps the first effort to harness our immune system to fight disease was that of William Jenner, almost 400 years ago. Jenner was a physician in England at a time when smallpox, a viral disease-causing fevers and pustules over the body and leading to deaths all over the world, was raging in England. The good doctor saw that milkmaids, exposed to a cousin virus in cows, called cowpox, didn't seem to get smallpox. Dr. Jenner's gardener had a nine-year-old son named James Phipps. With the cooperation of a milkmaid named Sarah Helmes who had cowpox pustules on her hand, some of the fluid from one of these pustules was inoculated into James' arm. Afterwards James had repeated exposures to persons with smallpox, but never got this highly contagious disease. Dr. Jenner, of course, wrote a paper on his research, "On the Origin of Vaccine Inoculation"

To be perfectly fair, the Chinese may have been the first to use a similar technique to protect people from death by smallpox. They took fluid from the blisters of victims and either inoculated it into the skin or gave it nasally to people who had not had smallpox yet and discovered that the smallpox these individuals got was much less likely to be fatal. This Chinese technique was done almost a millennium and a half before Jenner's experiment!

No-one who reads the history of the Americas can ignore the fact that smallpox, which had ravaged the rest of the world since its first appearance in Egyptian mummies, was lethal to native Americans after being introduced to the Americas in 1507.

So our immune systems, or lack thereof, have changed the course of history.

And just who is the enemy that our immune systems have been programmed to fight?? Mr. B.'s enemy was a bacterium which had crept through his defenses and had triggered an overwhelming response consisting of his fever, change in blood pressure and a racing heart, subjective feelings of unwellness and eventually confusion and unresponsiveness to his surroundings. Dr. Jenner was fighting a virus. Bacteria are one celled creatures, come in a variety of forms and shapes, can be seen under a microscope, live on our skin, in our intestines, mouth nose, vaginas and elsewhere and can be either friends or foes. (Lyme disease and pneumococcl pneumonia are two very dissimilar examples)

Viruses live and reproduce inside our body's cells and as in the case of the HIV virus, use our cells to produce more copies of themselves. Some viruses can cause our cells to go crazy and over time become malignant or cancerouus. The HPV virus, the agent provocateur of most cervical cancer, is such a virus.

Fungi and yeast, normally found in our vaginas, can have complicated life cycles, and you can see them too in your refrigerator hanging out on moldy cheese. Infections like Valley Fever (coccioidomycosis) and histoplasmosis are caused by geographically specific fungi.

Worms don't just live in the soil. A fair variety, with complex life cycles, have human hosts. Witness the sad story of the loving Jewish housewives migrating from Europe to 19th century America. In attempting to make traditional Gefiltefish treats for their families, they employed freshwater fish imported from the Great Lakes. In these raw fish lurked the formidable Diphyllobothrium, a species of fish tapeworm. Grandma cooks would taste gefilte fish preparations to assure quality, and unwittingly ingest the larva. When maturing into adulthood, these tapeworms can reach up to 25 meters. They can be asymptomatic, cause an upset stomach, or especially in the elderly cause megaloblastic anemia due to poor absorption of vitamin B12. Rarely they can also cause intestinal obstruction or gall bladder problems. (Jose A. Serpa, Miguel M. Cabata, A. Clinton White, Jr, Cestodes, Chapter 227 in Textbook of Pediatric Infectious Diseases, Eigth ed., James Cherry et al, ED, Elsevier, Philadelphia, Pa.2014)

Protozoa are one celled, sometimes free living, creatures and include the above-mentioned fungi. A few are even capable of invading our brains under select circumstances. Amoebae can cause an intestinal disease sometimes misidentified initially as ulcerative colitis, with bloody mucoid stools, weight loss and other complications including death. Trichominad flagellates can cause sexually transmitted vaginal and genital infection, and even get into the bladder. There are many other different varieties of the phylum protozoa, too numerous to even mention. However, the dreaded disease malaria is caused by one or more of five Geni of plasmodia, extracting a high morbidity and mortality in parts of the world tourists like to frequent.

Prions are the black hole of infectious agents. They are proteinacious agents capable of causing transmissible neurodegenerative diseases like kuru, a malady specific to the cannibalistic Fore tribe in Papua New Guinea. Thankfully, no more cases of kuru have occurred since the Kuru stopped eating cadaver brains.

It is important to realize that all of us are under constant attack from a myriad of these other creatures. Most diseases reflect some failure in our immune forces. For example, immune attacks against the cancer cells newly evolving in our bodies probably protect us constantly over the course of our lifetimes. You can think of most all cancers as our own cells turned rogue for a variety of reasons. And when the immune system gets confused and starts attacking the body it is supposed to be protecting, we can also see the emergence of autoimmune disease like lupus and perhaps type I diabetes. The process of becoming sick from a disease is very complex and influenced by our environments, life stresses, genetics and many other factors which we don't fully understand but suffice it to say that the warriors of our complex immune systems are at the ready to protect and defend.

The immune system is more complex than the armed forces! A brief overview of this complicated defense system is in order, since knowledge of its function is still evolving, especially with reference to changes in immune function as we age. Hold on for a brief look at a very complex system whose workings even modern science doesn't fully have a handle on yet.

The immune system has been divided into two main components, innate and acquired. The innate system is phylogenetically old, because even creatures in the primordial mud and oceans of the Cambrian period had enemies and therefore had to have some primitive sort of immune system.

The innate immune system, present at birth, recognizes microbes through pattern recognition receptors, zoning in to attack the groups of molecules that microbes, but not the host (human) possess. The analogy might be tracking an animal by the hoofprints or imprints in the soil made by that specific animal. When we consider innate immunity, whose components get to the scene of the invasion first, there are many parts. Physical barriers like the skin and the lining (mucosa) of the gastrointestinal tract, and even mucous itself, prevent microbes from slipping through the body's zone of defense, kind of a castle and moat arrangement. Enzymes in phagocytic cells like certain types of white blood cells (and epithelial cells) can injure or kill invaders. Serum proteins like those in the complement system are inflammation related and get quickly to the field of battle. Cells can have cell receptors, (toll-like receptors) which act like radar to sense micro-organisms and start a defensive response going. Specific cell types which are also part of the innate immune system (macrophages, mast cells, natural killer cells, innate lymphoid cells) have the duty of releasing cytokines and other types of inflammatory molecules that signal all the warriors linked to the battle (inflammation) to arrive NOW on the field of combat. And just like the Romans who eventually had to use barbarian tribes to help defend their borders, we have our own friendly bacteria and fungi, called the human biome, which live in and on the skin, intestines mouth, nose, and so forth and may be considered also a part of our innate immune system. Friendly bacteria, for instance, have their own defenses against alien bacteria trying to take over their cozy turf on the skin or in the large intestine. (40)(www.uptodate.com, Up to Date inc: Richard B. Johnston, Jr, MD, Senior Editor, Jordan. S. Orange, MD, PhD, Deputy Editor, Anna M. Feldweg, MD, Walters Kluwer)

The innate immune system is still being subject to research. WE have a lot more to learn about this rapid response system of ours which can respond quickly to a microbial or other invader, recognize the antigen (enemy) molecules broadly distributed in pathogens, and commence the battle till the more specific troops mobilize. Perhaps you could say that innate immunity is analogous to the marines, establishing a beachfront as other branches of the armed forces are being mobilized for more specific tasks.

The acquired immune system is a bit different. It is not fully active at birth, develops rapidly in infancy and childhood, and is environmentally more specific. It relies on two types of cells, the T and B lymphocytes. The T lymphocytes mature in and with the assistance of an organ called the thymus, which sits around the heart, and which is quite large in little babies. This system becomes much less effective as we age, and its senescence is under active investigation especially since the pandemic. Antibodies made by the interaction of the T and B cells, whether stimulated in response to the virus itself or induced by a vaccine, seem to be the key to controlling this (and other) pandemics.

A word about the complement system, whose function straddles both innate and adaptive immunity. The plasma proteins in the complement system both prepare invading bacteria for elimination and also themselves kill invading bacteria. They also alert components of the acquired immune system to come join the fight through activating an inflammatory response to pathogens. (41) (www.uptodate.com, UpToDate. Inc, Walters Kluwer. Complement pathways, M. Kathryn

Liscewski, PhD and John P. Atkinson, MD. Section Editors, E. Richard Stiehm, MD and Peter H. Schur, MD, Deputy Editor, Anna M Feldweg, MD)

Let's look more closely at the cells of the adaptive immune system. Luckily the adaptive immune system has primarily two main actors, T and B cells or lymphocytes. Both types are of course subdivided and also cooperate with the innate immune system. For example, phagocytosis, which is the ingesting and killing of an invading bacterium by a polymorphonuclear white blood cell swimming in the blood or nearing its functional maturity in the bone marrow, is greatly improved by the production of targeted antibodies by B cells. These antibodies are specific for the bacterium or virus doing the invading. Complicated? You bet! Those B cells that have been taught to make antibodies specific for one type of bacterium or virus will remember for their entire lives how to make those antibodies. So if you are now somewhere in your forties, and got chicken pox as a kid, or if you are sixty something and suffered through a week or more of measles as a child, your B cells will remember and start making antibodies to zap any wayward measles or chicken pox viruses you may be re-exposed to now. You will be protected by your immune system from getting another case of chicken pox or measles even after the passage of all those intervening years!

You can see that B cells must be initially exposed to an antigen, either from a germ or from a vaccine made from part of a germ, to develop this impressive lifelong memory.

So what do T lymphocytes do? They also are involved in the production of antibodies. Some kill cancer cells or virus infected cells (CD8+ lymphocytes)

Others (T4+ helper lymphocytes) help the B lymphocytes in their tasks in antibody production. Antibodies are the handcuffs of the immune system, which, when attached to an invading microbe allow the designated cells of the immune system to destroy the invader.

There are more T lymphocytes with specific tasks, but the interaction between the innate and adaptive immune systems and the specifics of intercommunication and cooperation between systems gets complicated and a lot more research is needed. Suffice it to say that this complex system always defends us against foreign invaders and against domestic terrorists such as damaged cells and nascient cancer.

Training, supply line and transportation are the next factors to consider. The immune system calls upon the spleen, thymus and lymphatic system for readying and mobilization of its forces

The thymus does its job of helping bring to mature function the T lymphocytes, and as mentioned, is positioned between the lungs, around the heart. By adolescence it has been largely replaced by fat, but it still seems to have responsibilities of a sort as we age.

The spleen, on the other hand, sits in the upper left back part of the abdomen and remains an important component of the immune system. It recycles old red blood cells and platelets and is important in fighting infections caused by bacteria like the pneumococcus, which can invade the lungs and even the central nervous system and elsewhere. People who have lost their spleens through accidents or due to certain diseases like sickle cell anemia are much more vulnerable to certain infections.

The lymphatic system (see vascular) has many roles, but a critical role relates to the transportation of immune cells to where they are needed. Lymph nodes filter waste and pathogens and assist T and B cells. You have probably noticed how your neck lymph nodes swell and even become tender when you have a viral or bacterial infection. Lymph vessels are thin-walled vessels that interdigitate with blood vessels to collect excess fluid between and around cells. The adjacent lymph nodes in their path filter out waste and harmful organisms. The lymph system has one foot in the camp of the vascular system. Drainage of the lymph system is into the subclavian veins on either side, with subsequent return to the right side of the heart. In this capacity, the lymphatic system helps to maintain fluid balance. The immune component of the lymphatic system, which also is comprised of the spleen and of the thymus, has to do with the interface between the innate and adaptive immune systems, and helping the T and B lymphocytes in their task of making specific antibodies to attack a targeted pathogen.

Additionally, lymph vessels also play a role in the transportation of fats.

Are you thoroughly confused yet?

What happens to a vibrant young immune system as it ages? As we age, our organ systems undergo changes which vary from individual to individual. Our immune systems are no exception. The exception is how little we know about changes in our immune systems as compared with, for example, changes in our kidneys or hearts!

However, there are a few general observations that really don't get down to causality but are helpful clinically.

- Some cancers increase in frequency and deadliness after age 65. Though there are many reasons for this, including more lifetime exposure to carcinogens, both the innate and adaptive immune systems are involved in early recognition of rogue cells headed toward cancer. Cancer also is not just one disease and immune responses may vary because of this and also the fact that most cancers don't develop overnight.
- Antibodies, those "handcuffing" agents produced by B-cells, are supposed to attack foreign invaders. As we age, autoantibodies, or self-directed antibodies, increase. The diseases autoantibodies cause, like rheumatoid arthritis and lupus, may present in a disguised form as weight loss, muscle aches and pains, and mental symptoms.
- Malnutrition may also contribute to the decline in immunity in the elderly. For example, vitamin D does more that strengthen bones and muscles. It also plays a role in immune function. But older folks' skins are less adept at playing their part in making vitamin D. Seniors generally are not out in the sun as much as younger folk either, or sunlight is an important component in making vitamin D.(42)(Antoine Azar, MD. Zuhair K. Bsallas, MD. Up To Date, Immune Function in Older adults, E. RichardStiehm, MD, Section Editor and Anna M. Feldweg, MD, Deputy Editor, Updated Sept 13, 2018)

    A thirty something woman, came in with a classic shingles rash, a bunch of tiny vesicles on a red base of skin which tracked from one of the nerves coming out from her spinal cord. She had chicken pox as a child, and the chicken pox virus, called varicella, had established a latent infection in one of her dorsal root or sensory ganglia. Ganglia, of course, are collections of nerve cell bodies in the peripheral nervous system coming from or going to the central nervous system. Some immunologic failure had roused the varicella virus from dormancy to travel down her sensory nerve to the nerve endings in the skin, in her case, of her right chest, causing her shingles rash. However, other than the fact that the rash was a bit ugly, she wasn't too alarmed. She felt no discomfort other than perhaps a slight itchiness, took the medication she was given and bounced back quickly.

A seventy something gentleman was seen for the same condition. However, in his case, he had such severe left chest pain prior to the appearance of his rash, that he was sent to the emergency room to be sure he wasn't having a heart attack. In the emergency room, doctors saw right before their eyes the evolution of a classis shingles rash. He also was given medication, but instead of bouncing back like the first patient, endured months of severe pain in the area of the rash, which was now long gone.

The difference in how mild a younger parson's shingles usually is compared with the devastation the varicella virus wrecks on an older person is in some way illustrative of the changes in a senior's immune system that weaken his or her fight against a variety of infections. In fact, the bacteria and viruses that can be so deadly in newborn babies, but rarely cause trouble in older children and adults, can attack the elderly with a frenzy. On the other hand, many elderly adults are immune to some types of influenza, a virus that mutates a lot, because the strain of influenza they had as a child has again become epidemic.

What to know about how the mature body handles infections

Older individuals often don't act as sick as they really are when they get infections. However, sometimes their symptoms are very confusing, can be severe, and very nonspecific too! For example, an older person with a serious or even life threatening infection can present with a fall, or increasing confusion, or if that person is suffering from dementia, it can be almost impossible to pinpoint early that serious illness is producing these confounding symptoms. Mature persons often don't have high fevers, don't complain of sweats., headaches and are used to body aches. Their immune systems are slower in responding to an invasion by pathogens (viruses, bacteria and so on) This means that an older person can be very ill before others recognize it. Medical personnel are generally aware of this phenomenon. If an older person has a temperature that is in the upper normal range for an infant's normal reading, say around 99 or 100 degrees Fahrenheit, his or her physician may begin a search for infection. Most older persons' normal temperature is often a degree or more lower than that of the average young adult. Should an older gentleman decide he is too tired to do his normal morning crossword puzzle when the daily paper arrives, or have an inexplicable fall, or if a nursing home patient who always enjoys her food unexpectedly refuse to eat, infection is one of the first diagnoses that needs to be ruled out. That infection may be an unsuspected pneumonia, or a raging kidney infection. (it of course could be something noninfectious like a silent heart attack).

Additionally, contact with grandchildren or other little rug rats can be an important source of infection. In fact, when a vaccine against the pneumococcus, a bacterium which causes a lot of pneumonia and other respirator infections, was introduced for infants, there was a statistical decline in pneumococcal infection in seniors, who had themselves not been vaccinated.

Because infections can be so stealthy in the elderly, vaccinations assume a new importance for older folk themselves. There is now a new reliable vaccine for shingles, two vaccines given in sequence for that nasty pneumococcus, and the tetanus, diphtheria and whooping cough vaccine (TDaP) is advisable every 10 years. If grandma is to take care of a new grandbaby, she should have a booster TDaP along with pregnant mom, dad and anyone else expected to be in close contact with the expected baby.

Look for amazing advances to be made in both the fields of immunology and of endocrinology in the near future!

CHAPTER 12

What to expect when you are your seventh decade of life

You are probably fully employed, and either looking ahead to retirement or making the decision to work past age 65.

If you have kept up with exercise and are eating a healthy diet, you may not notice too much of a change in your energy level.

Most women will be well past menopause, which usually happens in the early fifties. Hot flashes, palpitations, poor sleep and edgy nerves should be abating but you may notice some vaginal dryness, and perhaps a decreasing interest in sex. Or not. Breasts may be becoming slightly droopy as estrogen levels drop precipitously, especially if you were full breasted in youth.

Men may notice changes in the strength of erections and may be looking for the "little blue pill" to help out.

That tummy may be becoming a bit more pronounced, and men may notice that their urinary stream has thinned, perhaps they have some dribbling or note the need to urinate at night. Women, especially those with several pregnancies under their belt, may lose urine when they cough or laugh heartily. They may also notice an overwhelming tendency to void as they near a bathroom.

In both sexes, the same diet eaten in middle age will result in excess accumulation of fat as the need for calories decreases.

Somehow, caring for grandchildren, especially if more than one, becomes a bit more stressful than did caring for your own children.

Many retired people are able to do the things they had on their bucket lists, like traveling or perfecting a sport.

Communication between spouses can get better or worse, or both at the same time. As husbands retire, some want to take over household chores, which will either delight their wives, or frustrate them.

Finances take on a new dimension with retirement, and strategizing for the future a necessity.

Most people may have chronic health problems like high blood pressure or diabetes, that are manageable. Cancer may rear its ugly head and the disruption to plans and hopes as well as the physical consequences, are not really imaginable to those families not affected.

What to expect in the eighth decade of life

In your early seventies, there may not be much change from life in your sixties. But changes may require new methods of coping.

Digestion may become more of a problem. Acid reflex, intolerance to certain foods, especially fatty foods, may signal a need to be wiser about your diet. Alcohol also is metabolized differently, so care and moderation may be in your plan. Constipation and bloating, depending on your level of activity and your diet, may start to plague.

Urinary issues for both men and women may worsen. Men may find the need to use medications to urinate more easily. Women suffer more from both stress and urge incontinence, and may even notice what is called prolapse or a "falling down" of the bladder, urethra or sometimes the uterus, which may present as a "bulge" or "mass" down there.

Lubrication during sex and painful sex due to a dry fragile vaginal lining can be treated but many women are reluctant to discuss these problems or may no longer need to do so due to cessation of intercourse. Men find erectile dysfunction a common problem and may eventually find that the "little blue pill" and its mates no longer do the job.

Loss of energy may start to limit activity. It may just seem safer and easier to avoid going out and about. Vision may limit driving, especially at night, a general slowing down of reaction speed may cause anxiety about driving or engaging in other activities, competitive or not. Cataracts can be taken care of, and their occurrence may be noticed because oncoming headlights make night driving very difficult. Also more light is needed to see objects than was the case in earlier days,

Hearing also slowly decreases over time, especially for high pitched sounds. That means that a husband may not be ignoring his wife. She just normally has a higher pitch to her voice, so he truly cannot hear her! You can see the risk for marital issues arising here. Many people become aware of the onset of diminished hearing when they have trouble hearing in noisy places, such as busy restaurants, but still hear ok one on one in a quiet place.

Walking changes. The normal swing of one's arms becomes lessened. Painful joints may cause real pain and stiffness.

Falls can be a real issue. They have many reasons, of course. Balance is not as reliable, and once a person has fallen he or she becomes fearful of another fall. If one stops walking as much, the leg muscles become weaker, and a fall more likely.

Only a few brave people still want to travel the world!

However, for those who know that this life doesn't last forever, there is renewed attention to the things of the spirit. This can be a religious concern, a philosophical renewal, or for some, a state of resignation, of anxiety or of peace. Or perhaps all of the above. One's heritage also assumes increased importance. Some people may want to organize their own or their family's history to secure this information for posterity. A reexam of one's life is often a part of this state of introspection.

How about the ninth decade of life?

Forgetfulness may have manageable but present earlier in maturity, but is more pronounced in this decade. Most of the time, in spite of a person's fear of galloping Alzheimer's, forgetfulness is a normal feature of aging, if it is not progressive. Most people in their eighties will have "senior moments" when the word, or person's name just won't come when it should, although waiting a few minutes will help the desired word to pop out. On the other hand, rates of Alzheimer's or other types of dementing illness do increase during this decade.

Many people will have difficulty with activities that they had accomplished with ease in the prior decade. This may take the form of handing finances over to a child, spouse or friend. AS the decade progresses, tasks like showering and cooking become a greater challenge. Sometimes even getting out of bed is fraught with difficulty. For other folk, these chores and activities are not yet a problem. Chronic health problems become more a part of life though. Loss of teeth, especially molars, may place increasing restrictions on a person's diet, and so a balanced intake may warrant some creativity and nutritional knowledge on the part of caregivers. Hearing and vision may slowly decrease.

Though friends and family are still very important to physical, emotional and mental health, there are bound to be more losses and the greatest loss of all is that of a life partner. Medical problems escalate in the year after such a primal loss.

Turning inward, especially if accompanied by a further loss of energy, may mean more attention being paid to bygone days, which are seen sometimes in a golden haze, of sometimes as times of privation.

Spiritual concerns rise in importance in most people. Those with belief find consolation which can be of great importance.

Many people in the ninth decade of life, living with the physical restrictions imposed by aging, can actually enjoy the little things in life that they didn't have time for in their younger days. They can be a real support to their families and friends by listening, giving objective advice when solicited, just by being there. Happy people tend to stay happy into old age, and can serve a reassuring role just by their gratitude for what younger people may overlook.

Okay, the tenth decade!

People who have made it this far can be a lot of fun! They may possess good genes, usually have a positive outlook, and when they decide to, can tell interesting stories.

Generally, they need some help with routine activities, but not always. Some maintain a fierce independence. Nonetheless, there is still a sense that this life will end, so preparation is a good idea.. Seeing and hearing can be a real issue, and no one likes to wear hearing aides all the time. Nasty little bodily problems like incontinence, constipation, poor mobility, even passing gas just have to be lived with. As taste and smell decline, a juicy steak isn't in the cards. The skin is much more fragile, and infections last longer and can be much more dangerous.

For quite a few, medication use can paradoxically decline. Sleep cycles can either become irregular or sleep can greatly increase as a percentage of one's day.

And Alzheimer's becomes more prevalent, along with a decline in other random organs.

There is a wide splay in the functioning of quite people, depending on lifelong health practices, diet, genetics, social support and one's innate glass-full or empty personality.

Beyond the tenth decade

WE definitely are in uncharted territory here. But 100 year old s compete in the Senior Olympics, some still work, and then there is the French Nun who held the honor of being the authenticated oldest person in the world. She survived Covid. The story is that when asked at age 116 or so about when she planned to retire, she quipped "In this job (as a religious) we don't get to retire". So yes, that impish sense of humor was there till the end!